Fibromyalgia Handboook

Based on Marta's Recovery

Maribel Ortells

Author: Maribel Ortells
Design and layout: Soul Goes Social, S.L.
Copyright© 2011 Vicente Estupiñá and Maribel Ortells

First edition of this infoproduct: November 2011

Translation: Estela Miralles
ISBN-10 : 1985092662
ISBN-13: 978-1985092662

CONTENTS

Testimonials 6

  Hi, I am Marta................ 7

  I'm Maribel, Marta's mother 11

  Coincidences 27

Fibromyalgia 29

  What is it? 30

  Symptoms and Syndromes 30

  Why does it appear and its causes 37

What is Candidiasis? 41

The Diet 55

  Basic Recommendations.. 56

Nutrition 60

  Fruits 62

  Calcium 62

  Sugar and refined products 63

  The other face of dairy products 64

  Algae 68

  Millet 72

  Magnesium 74

  Umeboshi 75

  Kuzu 76

  Sugar 78

Bowel Hypersensitivity.... 81

  The importance of Carbohydrates 84

  The Acid/Alkaline Balance 86

  Acid/Alkaline Foods 87

Our Proposal 89

  Allergies and other Diseases 90

  Beneficial, Neutral and Harmful Foods 90

  Recommendations 91

    Cereals as source of life ... 92

  Diet sample for all Blood Groups 95

Blood Group 101

  Group "0" 102

  Group "A" 111

  Group "B" 120

  Group "AB" 130

  Marta's advise 139

  Coffee 140

  Tobacco 141

Recipes 142

Author 153

Testimonials

HI, I AM MARTA

I´d like to tell you my story, I believe a lot of people will identify with it, because people who suffer this illness feel the same way, more or less.

Everything started about three years ago, well, the truth is that it really started sooner, but we began to see it clearly later on. Coming back home after a handball game, all of us usually felt tired, but I always was exhausted, more than the rest of the team. One day, on a WiseMen's play, I participated as a page-boy, I remember going home afterwards, I felt like I wasn't going to be able to make it there because of the enormous pain I was feeling on my legs, and because I was feeling so terribly tired.

All these symptoms puzzled us, my parents and me, because it wasn´t normal that a girl my age often asked for a wheelchair because I couldn´t move. Some people told me that I was lazy, I had to hear that, even from some teachers and doctors.

My mother was starting to think that it could be fibromyalgia, but we had little information about it, so we decided to go to the hospital. After a whole week of stay there, the doctors finally confirmed that it was in fact fibromyalgia. At first, I didn´t know how to react because I had never heard that word before, but a month went by and I started to wish I had never heard about this illness, because I realized that it was going to last a lifetime and if I had to assume this illness, I would have to put up with mockery coming from people all around me.

When I thought my life was coming to an end, and considered I would never be able to live as a normal human being again, my mom found a book that talked about blood groups.   We had already tried many things, so why not try one more? We had nothing to lose.   At first, it was hard to get used to the diet, we started trying out different types of food, and the truth is that it didn't taste very good.   Months passed by, and I could walk again and do things just like all the rest, so we decided to continue with the diet.

When I saw that I could run again, without having any contractures or without getting any broken fibers, I suddenly became a happier girl, I was happy before then, but I felt like now I had a greater desire to live, to travel, or to go out with my friends at night.

At this moment, I feel very proud about all my parents and my friends have done for me: they all decided to eat the same food I ate, just to make it easier for me. I will always be grateful to them for that.

I hope this book will help all the people who suffer this illness around the world, to   help them enjoy again with all the hopes they had before, and they possibly lost by now.

My parents have decided to explain all this in a book in order to help out, and to make sure nobody has to suffer as much as I have, and also   to   show everybody, including doctors, that there is a solution to fibromyalgia.   I hope all of them who suffer now will soon get better.

I also believe that talking about it helps to improve, I have experienced this myself.   Once, at school, we had to do an oral presentation in front of the class, we had to talk during four minutes about a theme of our own choice.

After consulting with my mother, I decided that fibromyalgia was a theme I knew something about. I practiced at home about what I was going to say about it, and it seemed like I had everything under control, but nobody was to know what was just about to happen.

It was my turn, and I went out to the blackboard, in front of all my classmates. Everything seemed to go just fine, until just a moment after explaining what fibromyalgia was, about all the people affected by it around the world, and the symptoms caused by this illness, the moment arrived when I had to confess in front of everybody that two years sooner, I was the one diagnosticated with fibromyalgia. Just then, I started to notice that words couldn´t come out from my mouth, and I felt like I run out of air, suddenly I started to cry, and I wasn´t able to stop. All my classmates looked at me, feeling helpless, not knowing what to do, and I heard my teacher telling me to breath and calm down.

It was then when I really realized how much I had suffered, and how ill I could have been. I also thought about my parents, and how much they had suffered because of me. It was like, all of a sudden, something came out, something that had been deeply hidden inside of me. The truth is that I was surprised, I felt relaxed and it made me feel great. With my friends help, I could continue and finish my story, a story I had never had the courage to share with anyone before.

My parents have worked really hard to make sure other people who suffer fibromyalgia listen to them and follow their advise.   I thank them for their constant fight. And, to all the people who suffer it, I wish to tell them that with perseverance, patience, and willpower, they can overcome it, just the way I did.

Kisses,

Marta

I'M MARIBEL, MARTA'S MOTHER

I'm writing this letter in Borriol, Castellon, a small village with a population of about five thousand.

Actually, neither my husband nor I come from Borriol, my husband was born in Portell de Morella, a village in the interior mountain range of Castellon, and I am from Vila Real, a city near Castellon, but for the last 18 years, our lives have turned around Borriol.
Our daughters were born here, and they couldn't even think about living anywhere else.

Here, children play on the street, and we know almost everybody, it's an advantage of living in a small village; ours is placed at only 7 Km from Castellon, and in a small period of 15 minutes, approximately, you can be at the capital and enjoy all of its advantages.

Everything about health and nutrition has always been of our interest, and every week we buy magazines about these matters. We had no idea that in the near future this knowledge was going to be of great assistance to us, in order to help our daughter to recuperate her health and her happiness, and as a consecuence, to help our entire family.

I have two daughters, Aranxa, 17 years old, and Marta, 14 years old. Aranxa has quite serious allergies, which in more than one occasion have taken us to the hospital's emergency with anaphylactic shock, and for this reason we started to investigate the ways to improve her allergies.

I, their mother, also have my own problem. Ever since I was a little girl, I've had problems of irritable bowel, all people who have this problem surely know what I'm talking about, and almost all people with fibromyalgia also suffer this illness.

And at last, I get to our main character, for better of for worse, Marta.

Marta was born on the 29th December 1990, she was a quiet and good baby, but when she was hungry, her father had to walk her around the house to calm her down until the feeding bottle was ready. She has always been very loving and friendly, and also tender and caring towards her friends, animals, and for everything in general, and very responsible with all her commitments.

She has long, brown hair, with honey-coloured eyes, she is constantly worried about looking cool, but always with her personal touch.

Looking back into Marta's life, I realize that

when she was only 3 years old, she started having symptoms of this illness.   At that age, when she got out of the nursery, her eyes were always dirty because she was constantly touching them.   At first, I argued with her about it, until I realized it wasn't just a bad habit but a reaction to something that wasn't going well.   The pediatrician confirmed that Marta constantly touched her eyes because they were dry, and she applied her saliva on them to calm down that sensation of dryness.

When she was 5 years old, Marta's pain problems began.

Marta was a girl full of life, she liked playing with her friends, running, jumping, just like the rest of the kids.   But, when she got home, she always complained about the pain on her feet.   At first, we didn't pay too much attention, but weeks went by, and we saw the pain didn't go away, so her pediatrician sent us directly to the traumatologist.

The traumatologist did x-ray examinations that revealed why her feet hurt, her heels were very fragile due to decalcification and he prescribed her an anti-inflammatory and an analgesic, and also some gel insoles to cushion her body weight on every step she took.

We tried all these things, but Marta's pain continued; we went shopping and as soon as she got a chance, she sat down, because her feet hurt and she needed to sit down to rest.

When she was 9 years old, she started having pain on her knees; they gave her more anti-inflammatory pills and more analgesics to calm down her pain. The truth is that all those pills didn't work at all, but at that moment, we couldn't and didn't know what else to do.

When she was 10 years old, the traumatologist decided to plaster Marta's leg, to see if the pain disappeared, but when he took it off, after a whole month, nothing had changed. And the worst was yet to come.

On April 2002, Marta was playing handball with the school team, and when she got home she could barely go up the stairs, she was so tired it was impossible.

Marta said that she was more tired then usual, so we took her to the doctor, he did a blood test that revealed that Marta had no apparent problems, so the doctor attributed it all to the springtime.

Summertime helped a little, she could sleep more and rest in the afternoon.

We noticed that whenever she went out, riding

her bicycle or swimming with her friends, she felt quite tired, but she is strong, and she always tried not to stop moving.

The time came to get back to school, and we didn't know what would happen.

In October, she had suffered a hamstring on her leg, she was only playing with her friends, her teacher called us at home, so we could go pick her up at school. She told us she didn't know what had happened, she was playing around and suddenly she simply couldn't walk because of the pain she felt.

The doctor said it was just a muscle strain, to take an analgesic and with a few days of rest it would disappear, but the days passed by and she didn't get any better. A more exhaustive exploration done by the traumatologist showed that what she really had was not a muscle strain, but a hamstring. They had to put a bandage on and keep her home with absolute rest.

Two weeks later, the hamstring was on the other leg, while she was going up the stairs. Then the traumatologist decided to do some clinical tests to see if she had some rheuma in her blood and see if that was the cause of all her problems. The tests were all perfect.

Contractures started to appear all over her body, she couldn't even carry her school bag because she had so much pain on her shoulder blades and her arms that it was impossible for her to carry it. At that moment, I decided to go with Marta to school everyday, and I personally carried her bag, in order to avoid all the pain on her back and arms.

Doing any exercise was an ordeal for her because her whole body hurt. We were lucky with her sports teacher, he understood that she was not just trying to avoid doing some sport, and he suggested her to do only what she could without forcing her body.

In November, the problems went on. The pediatrician kept saying that it was the flu. I believed her at first, but three weeks later, I thought that it was very doubtful and suspicious that she still had the flu.

We started with the blood tests, x-rays, ultrasounds, tacs, but all we tried didn't show anything not normal, and Marta felt worse each day. At this moment, the traumatologist told us he didn't know why Marta had so much pain and contractures and that he couldn't do anything else for her, because he was totally lost, he didn't know what other tests he could do.

In December the problem got worse because Marta fell asleep on the sofa when she came back from school, she sweated a lot   and there was no way to wake her up.

At school, there was a teacher who laughed down at her all the time, in front of all her friends, saying that her problem was that she didn't want to work and she wanted to pass without any effort.   These comments really hurt Marta's feelings, she couldn't understand why nobody believed that she was really suffering with terrible pain all over her body.

On December the 15th, Marta told me   she couldn't go to school, she could barely walk and she couldn't sit down on the chair neither, the pain was beyong all bearing.   The pain was so bad, she couldn't even hold the pencil or open a plastic bag.

At the time, Marta took some ibuprofen every four hours, but with no results.

Christmas came and it was difficult to bear, for Marta and for all of us, her family.   Watching her suffering on the sofa, and at the same time fighting because she wanted to go out with her friends.   It was absolutely terrible.

On the Wisemen Day's Eve, she was performing on a play as a Page Boy and she could barely walk, but she is very stubborn and when she wants something, she fights for it to the end.   That day was terrible, taking painkillers every four hours and not getting better at all.

As a consecuence, the Wisemen Day she couldn't even get out of bed to see her presents, she was so tired with fatigue and pain that it was a pity to see her, and it was at that time when we started to worry very seriously.

On Jannuary the 8th 2003, she had a strong headache and pain on her neck and back, she couldn't sleep more than three hours in a row at night, and she couldn't get out of bed. We took her to emergencies with all the test and x-rays we had done previously to her, everything was ok, they told us to keep taking analgesics and they sent her home.

Three days later, we went there again, and I told them if they could consider the possibility of her having fibromyalgia. We had been looking it up on internet and the symptoms Marta had were exactly as the symptoms explained on internet for fibromyalgia patients. They decided to get her into the hospital.

We stayed at the hospital for a week, they did all kinds of tests, but of course, they were all normal, and the pediatrician told us that it was, in effect, juvenile fibromyalgia, he gave her an aspirin and sent her home again, saying that having fibromyalgia was nothing too serious.

We were shocked, and we told him that we had already been giving her aspirin for a long time, and even stronger painkillers, but she didn't get any better.

The pediatrician didn't know what to say, he recognized he had no idea about fibromyalgia, and let alone that it can happen to such a young person.

We returned home.   Marta couldn't even go to school, the pain didn't let her sleep and she got no rest, her body got weaker, and her pain and general fatigue only got worse.

In March, we went to the Clinical Hospital in Barcelona, there we were attended by a fantastic team who tried their best to help us with antidepressants, relaxants, and sleeping pills. Each trip to Barcelona was a big personal effort that caused her to be several days in bed due to all the pain resulting from it.

As days went by, Marta felt even worse, due to the pills she was always falling asleep, some days she couldn't even talk, and let alone get our of bed, and even then we came along with some doctor who said that she was causing all that herself, just to get attention. These words left Marta completely torn, she couldn't understand how they could tell her something like that. All she wanted was to get well, and to be able to go out, play and run with her friends.

It was in the month of May when I discovered the book: "Blood groups and Nutrition" by doctor Peter

D'Adamo and Catherine Whitney.

We started reading it and, to our surprise, we discovered that it talked about chronic fatigue and the way, not to cure it, but about how to improve the lives of those patients who suffer it.

Also, at that time, in a health food store we heard about another book "Balance through Nutrition" by doctor Olga Cuevas Fernandez. It helped us to understand a lot of theories that we had and were wrong about nutrition, and it would become the foundation of Marta's recovery.

Beginning with the diet was very complicated, because it meant a radical change in the type of food we ate at home until then, but we had to try.

The first week was very hard, apart from the change of food, Marta suffered an aggravation, with a lot of pain all over her body. We talked with a naturalist physician, and he told us it was normal, he even assured us that the aggravation meant that her body was cleansing and in a few days all the symptoms would start to disappear. Actually, by the end of the second week, Marta stopped asking for sleeping pills, she forgot to take it one day, and she slept all night long.

We also stopped giving her the analgesics she was taking, and this was a decision taken by my husband and I, as we realized that, so far, they had not been positive on improving the illness, and being our sole responsibility , we decided not to give them to her anymore. I must say it was the best decision we could have taken, because right afterwards, we saw that Marta was more awake and she felt more active to do things like reading or talking.

The last week of the school year, and after a few months with her new eating habits, she returned to school, after a five month period during which she had not been able to assist regularly, and we saw that her body responded perfectly.

We started to combine the diet with regular massages, done by a physiotherapist, who told us that Marta's back had so many contractures that she would need several months to notice any improvement.

After three weeks of diet, the contractures almost disappeared, the physiotherapist was surprised, he didn't expect to see such a quick recovery.

By the end of July, we went to the Clinical Hospital in Barcelona again, and after doing a general check up, they couldn't believe what they were seeing, when they explored her back, the contractures had almost disappeared, and her physical and emotional appearance was great.

Marta was not feeling sleepy all day, and she didn't suffer with pain all over her body.   She now knows all she has to do is eat natural food and food which is beneficial for her illness. It cost a lot of crying, sacrifice and arguments with her, but she can see by herself that if someday she eats food which is not allowed, she feels tired and the pain and contractures come back.

Two years have gone by since we started with her problems in September 2002, but now, two years later, Marta continues with her diet and she is living a totally normal life, she has learned how to eat   without any problems, but only food which benefits her body.

The whole family is following this diet and we all feel great, I would say that much better then before. Personally, since I follow this type of diet, a healthy diet I believe, all the digestive problems and the irritable bowel problems I used to suffer are totally gone.

I forgot to say that Marta also suffered with irritable bowel since she was born, and nowadays that's all in the past, just like her illness. Another problem she had was that twice or three times a year she had sinusitis with headaches and lots of mucus, and since she stopped drinking milk, this has also disappeared.

Nowadays, Marta plays handball, goes to High School and goes out with her friends, she even goes to parties when it's necessary and all this is possible because she is keeping up with this way of nutrition. She is not taking any medicines and she's even stronger and healthier than some of her friends.

In this book, we want to share our experience with all the patients who suffer this terrible disease, and give them our support.   We know that many of these patients feel alone and rejected by their family, who think they complain only to get some attention, and by some doctors, who send them to the psychologist and end up with a "troublesome" patient to whom they don't know what to say, or how to treat.

During the last year, we have talked with many affected people, almost all of them have gone through back, wrist, or feet surgery. None of them have noticed any improvement with surgery, on the contrary, they have usually noticed a pain aggravation.

From here, we ask for more support and understanding towards people with fibromyalgia.

With the kind of diet people are now following, this and many other diseases like rheumatism, osteoporosis, sclerosis and similar, will be a plague in a very near future, because so much fat, sugar and junk food are attacking our bodies, making them weak and leaving them without any defenses. We must change to a healthy and well-balanced diet.

I would like to tell you, one of the many experiences I have lived ever since Marta became ill, it happened a few months ago.

It was at the end of March, Marta started to complain with abdominal pain, at first it wasn't very sharp or strong, but it hurt more each day, so we decided to visit her doctor; in the first check up, he didn't know what to tell us, and he prescribed her a syrup to discard a gas accumulation.

The pain got stronger, and in a second visit, he sent us to the hospital, thinking it might be appendicitis.

At the hospital, as we explained her symptoms, they thought it could possibly be appendicitis, but they had to make sure by doing some tests and x-rays, which as usual, turned out to be normal.

They prescribed her an abdominal relaxant and waited for her evolution. Days went by and our visits to emergencies went up to four, and we still didn't know the reason that caused this stomachache.

We decided to visit an urologist, friend of the family. During his check up, he found no reason for the pain, the appendix was not swollen, neither were the kidneys, so he decided to do an abdominal tac to discard any unexpected complication.

The tac didn't show anything strange, that calmed us down, but the pain persisted.

We returned to emergencies, and the only thing they thought to see in the tac was a feces accumulation in Marta's bowel, but I could not believe it, considering her problem with irritable bowel had always caused her to have frequent diahrrea.

I must say that the pain stopped, just as quickly as it had appeared, and until recently, we didn't know why.

Marta used to take magnesium pills, three each day, and following our intuition, we decided to have her stop taking them, and instead of pills, we gave her the magnesium in blisters. One month ago, we decided to give her the magnesium pills again, and the pain returned. It was clear to us, the pills had been the cause, because they contained a bigger concentration of that mineral than she could assimilate, it was too much magnesium for her, and her bowel rejected it causing the pain, she stopped taking them or she took only one pill a day, and the pain disappeared.

Sometimes, it's our own body who tells us that something is going wrong, and if we pay it enough attention, we can solve many problems which may have their origin in something as simple as the food we eat everyday, which is harming us without us knowing it.

The human body is wise, we must only listen to it. Doing this, we can assure our daughter Marta has recovered. That's exactly what I wish for all of you.

Maribel Ortells
(Borriol. January 2005)

COINCIDENCES

Life is made up with small coincidences that fill our day to day with unexpected surprises, and there is no better example than our own experience.

In it, the name of Marta plays an essential role due to a series of very curious coincidences:

-We used different sources to prepare and make this handbook, among them, Dr. D'Adamo's book, whose wife's name is Marta.

-Marta is also the name of the cooperating partner of Dr. Cuevas.

-And finally, closing the circle of women's names, our daughter's name is also Marta.

We would like to refer to an ancient myth that has as heroine a woman called Marta.

There is a medieval legend that tells about a battle that Santa Marta fought against a fearsome dragon, and tells us how the saint escaped unharmed dominating that mythological creature. The story tells that Santa Marta travelled to Marseille and with the help of a book dripped in oil and her willpower, she was able to defeat and submit the terrible beast. Santa Marta's image is always accompanied with a book and at times, tied by a chain, is also present the submitted dragon.

Our daughter Marta also put all her determination to defeat the bad thing that was not allowing her to live a normal life, fibromyalgia. Maybe this legend hides a bit of truth among its lines full of fantasy and what it wants to tell us is that people, just like Marta, can overcome all the obstacles they find along the way.

FIBROMYALGIA

WHAT IS IT?

Fibromyalgia is a chronic rheumatical disease also known as the invisible disease: it can't be detected through any x-ray or clinical test. The patients that suffer it don't show any visible alteration, even though they have a lot of symptoms: chronic pain in different parts of the body, which take them to stillness, muscle contractures in extremities, back, neck and cervicals, bone weakness (they often suffer with scoliosis, slipped disc, and rheumatical problems) general tiredness, sleep disorders, insomnia, irritable bowel syndrome, dizziness, tingling on extremities, memory and concentration difficulty... the only objective diagnosed proof for fibromyalgia is the pressure in 18 body points that result abnormally painful when pressured.

SYMPTOMS AND SYNDROMES ASSOCIATED TO FIBROMYALGIA

Apart from pain and exhaustion, there are a number of symptoms/syndromes generally related to fibromyalgia. Just like the pain and the exhaustion, the harshness of these symptoms/syndromes tends to increase and decrease, due to this reasons, the discomfort caused to the patients changes according to its severity. In general, patients with fibromyalgia suffer with one or more of the following usual symptoms:

STIFFNESS

Apart from the pain, their body stiffness can represent an oppressive problem for people with fibromyalgia. This stiffness usually appears early in the morning, after a period sitting down or standing still for a while, after a change of temperature or relative humidity.

INCREASE OF FACE AND HEADACHES

Face / headaches are a regular result from extremely stiff neck or shoulder muscles, transmitting the pain upwards. They can also come along with the disfunction of a temporomandibular joint (also known as TMJ), a condition which affects approximately one third of the patients with fibromyalgia and affects the articulations of the jaws and their corresponding muscles.

SLEEP DISORDERS

Even sleeping enough hours, patients with fibromyalgia can wake up feeling tired, as if they hadn't gotten enough sleep. On another hand, they can have problems trying to fall asleep or to stay asleep. We don't know the reasons why fibromyalgia causes sleep not to be relaxing enough, or causes other sleep disorders. But, the first investigations done in sleep laboratories about fibromyalgia, showed interruptions in the deepest sleep stage (the delta stage) on some patients with fibromyalgia.

COGNITIVE DISORDERS

People with fibromyalgia inform about a variety of cognitive symptoms that change day by day. These include trouble to concentrate, mental slowness, "fibro-fog", memory lapses, trouble to remember words/names and an overwhelming feeling whenever they have different things to do all at once.

ABDOMINAL DISCOMFORT

Many people with fibromyalgia experience digestive disorders, abdominal pain, flatulence, constipation and/or diarrhea. These symptoms are known together as "Irritable bowel syndrome" (IBS). In addition, some patients have trouble to pass food, which according to investigations is a result of objective abnormalities in the smooth muscle found in the esophagus.

GENITOURINARY PROBLEMS

It is possible that patients with fibromyalgia complain of increase in frequency or urgency to urinate, without suffering a bladder infection.

Some patients may also present a more chronic condition such as a painful inflammation of the bladder walls, which is know as *intestinal cystitis* (IC). In women, fibromyalgia can cause menstrual periods to be more painful and fibromyalgia's symptoms are worse during those days.   Also in women, we can find other conditions, such as vulvar vestibulitis or vulvodynia, recognized by the pain caused in the vulvar area and pain during intercourse.

PARESTHESIA

Sometimes the SMF is associated with numbness or tingling (for example, in hands and feet). Also known as paresthesia, which can be described as a feeling of itching and burning.

HYPERSENSITIVE MYOFASCIAL POINTS

An important number of patients with fibromyalgia have a neuromuscular condition known as myofascial pain syndrome (MPS) in which we find some extremely painful points (hypersensitive points) expanded in shrunken strips in muscles or other connective tissues, many times due to an injury resulting from repeated movements, incorrect posture during a long period of time, or from illness.   They are not only very painful, but they transmit the pain to other parts of the body in many predictable ways.

Unlike fibromyalgia's ways to affect the body, MPS is a condition located in very specific areas, often in neck, shoulders or waist.TMJ is considered a form of this syndrome.

CHEST SYMPTOMS

Fibromyalgia patients who participate in activities which force them to bend forward (for example, typewriting, sitting on a desk, working with a computer, being in a production line, etc), often have peculiar problems with pain on their chest or upper body parts, known as chest pains or disfunctions.

Often, these pains come with panting for breath and postural problems. Some patients can also present a condition called "costochondralgia" (also know as costochondritis), which is a muscular pain were the ribs meet the breastbone, sometimes this is confused with a heart disease. People with fibromyalgia are sensitive to a generally asymptomatic heart condition called "mitral valve prolapse"(MVP) in which one of the heart valves gets swollen during a beat, causing a click or murmur. Generaly, MVP is not a cause for concern in fibromyalgia patients, unless there is another heart condition.

Note: Any person who experiences chest pain, must always and immediately consult a physician.

IMBALANCE

Fibromyalgia patients can experience problems of imbalance due to a series of reasons. Considering we believe that fibromyalgia affects the eye's follow-up skeletal muscles, they can experience nausea or "visual confusion" when they drive a car, read a book or follow objects with their sight. Difficulties with the smooth muscles of the eye can also cause other focus problems.

It could also happen that having weak muscles, or hypersensitive points in the neck, a malfunction of TMJ can produce imbalance. Investigations at the John Hopkins Medical Center have also proved that some fibromyalgia patients have a condition known as "Hypotension of neurological origin" which causes, when they stand up, a decrease in blood pressure and heart rate, causing dizziness, nausea, and problems to think clearly.

LEGS SENSIBILITY
Sometimes, some fibromyalgia patients show a neurological disorder known as "restless legs syndrome" (RLS). This condition is characterized by an uncontrollable impulse to move their legs, mostly when resting and relaxing. A recent study revealed that a 31% of fibromyalgia patients have RLS. This syndrome can also produce periodical movements of the extremities while sleeping "periodic limb movement syndrome"(PLMS) which can be very annoying to the patient and to his mate.

SENSE HYPERSENSITIVITY/ ALLERGIC SYMPTOMS
Hypersensitivity to light, sound, touch and smell is usual in fibromyalgia patients, and we believe that it is due to an excess of surveillance of the nervous system. Besides, some people with fibromyalgia can have chills or feel cold while other people feel fine; or

they may feel hot while others don't. They can suffer reactions similar to allergies towards a number of substances which come with itching and rash, or sometimes the patients experience a form of non-allergic rhinitis recognized by cold, nose excretions and pain in the nasal sinuses, but without immunological reactions which appear in allergic conditions. But, when such symptoms appear, there is normally no response from the immune system as it usually happens in a real allergic reaction.

SKIN PROBLEMS

Annoying symptoms, like itching, dryness or stains, may come along with fibromyalgia. Patients with fibromyalgia can also experience a strange sensation, particularly in their extremities, on their fingers. Often, their ring doesn't fit. Nevertheless, this type of swelling is not arthritis, but it is a located abnormality of fibromyalgia which cause is unknown.

DEPRESSION AND ANXIETY

Often, fibromyalgia patients are wrongly diagnosed with depression and anxiety disorders, ("you are making it all up"), research has repeatedly shown that fibromyalgia is not a form of depression or hypochondria. However, when depression or anxiety come with fibromyalgia, it's very important to treat them, considering these conditions might aggravate fibromyalgia and interfere with the successful handling of its symptoms.

(1) Extract from an article of National Fibromyalgia Partnership

WHY DOES IT APPEAR AND ITS CAUSES

According to doctors D'Adamo/Catherine Whitney, in their book- "Blood Groups and Nutrition":

"Sometimes even though the symptoms of some autoimmune diseases like chronic fatigue and fibromyalgia are disguised as a virus of a disease of the immune system, the most probable cause of its origin is a problem of a poor metabolism of the liver".

Acording to Dr. Olga Cuevas in her book- "Balance through Nutrition":

"In some autoimmune diseases, like fibromyalgia, the problem of poor metabolism of the liver is originated in the intestinal walls, these are permeable to allow the pass of nutrients to the blood;   the intestinal barrier is not perfect and it leaves it easy for some "intruders" to get in, which doesn't suppose a problem for most individuals".

Real problems start when the intestinal walls get swollen and become hyperpermeable.   That is to say, people who due to genetic reasons have their intestinal walls thinner than normal or due to other causes that we will talk about later on, they get the intestinal walls swollen during the assimilation process; and besides nutrients, other waste substances and toxic food get through their intestinal walls.   These arrive to the liver and kidneys for their disposal, being overwhelmed by them.   The immune system gets then into action, and it considers them enemies declaring them a war.

This brings a vitamin wear in the body and toxic substances are produced which can accumulate in different parts of the body, producing injuries to different levels (in bones, in muscles and neuromuscular)".

Among other causes that can cause intestinal swelling and hyperpermeability we can find:

> Intake of food not allowed according to our blood group. According to doctor D'Adamo, we can find in food and bacteria, some molecules called lectins with binding properties, when lectins go through the intestinal walls and get to the blood, they have a reaction with certain blood components and they produce clumps.
> A 95% of the lectins that we absorb from our diet, are refused by the body, but at least 5% (more for hyperpermeable bowels) get to the blood, "attack" the red and white blood cells, and cause many problems especially related with the immune system.
> In the digestive tract, the lectins often create a Swelling of the mucous membrane and its binding action may seem a food intolerance.
> The real solution to many autoimmune diseases is doing a diet that cleanses the body, reinforces the bowels and increases our defenses.

Another important cause for intestinal hyperpermeability are treatments with steroids and non-steroid antiinflammatories, including aspirin. These medicines swell the intestinal walls and cause the widening of the cell spaces. Abnormal intestinal flora, produced mostly by the abuse of antibiotics that destroy the bacterial flora and allow the proliferation of yeasts and harmful fungi.
The abuse of animal products, fats, dairy products and the intake of little fiber, which favours the development of coli bacteria, causing putrefaction in detriment of the beneficial acidophils.
Substances that irritate the digestive tract, like tobacco, alcohol, coffee, additives, spices, sugar, ...

Other causes (see chapter about intestinal hyperpermeability).

HOW DOES IT AFFECT OUR BODY

When the bowel gets swollen, it doesn't absorb the nutrients correctly, and it may cause gas, swelling, abdominal pain, indigestion, constipation or diarrhea.

Proteins transported may be injured and then nutritient deficiency appears, like calcium deficiency (in fibromyalgia patients we find bone weakness and derived problems like scoliosis, back problems, osteoporosis, etc).

Another important deficiency is that of magnesium, which produces muscle contractures all over the body, specially on back, neck and extremities (this explains the 18 body parts that result abnormally painful when pressed).

It can also produce other deficiencies of copper, zinc or selenium causing general fatigue which, along with the pain, keeps the patient from getting a good night sleep and produces him a lack of concentration and bad memory.

TREATMENT WITH TRADITIONAL AND NATURAL MEDICINE
In cases of fibromyalgia, present medicine prescribes analgesics, muscle relaxants and anti-depressants.

Other alternative medicines act with different remedies like acupuncture, physiotherapy or psychology. But all these remedies are used once the problem is already manifest.

We are going to try to intercept the problem from its foundation, with a nutrition that cleans the body and increases our defenses. Only that way we'll start the cure.

What is Candidiasis ?

WHAT IS CANDIDIASIS?

I believe that many diseases have their start with this illness, called Candidiasis, it's very important to understand what it is and which are its symptoms in order to do what's necessary and to follow an appropriate diet to control it.

Candidiasis is an infection caused by a yeast of the Candidas family. There are about 150 different Candidas species, like Kruse Candida, Glabrata Candida, Tropicalis Candida, Parapsilosis Candida, etc. However, the most commonly found in our body is the Albicans Candida.

Yeasts are present in all of us shortly after birth, and they live in harmony with us. They are found in our skin, in our digestive system and in our genitourinary system. Their function is to absorb a certain quantity of heavy metals to prevent their entrance in our blood, they help us to degrade badly digested carbohydrates leftovers, and these, along with bacteria, maintain our intestinal balance and ph balance.

The intestinal and vaginal flora, along with the immune system, help us to maintain these yeasts under control.

Nevertheless, there are a series of factors that can put down our immune system, and unbalance our intestinal flora, causing an excessive growth of these yeasts, and therefore, the disease.

These factors are:

Excess of sugar or refined carbohydrates: These are the main nourishment for candidas. Apart from nourishing them directly, sugar and refined flour increase the glucose levels in blood, through which we can also nourish them.

Regular intake of tap water: Chlorine destroys intestinal flora, and fluoride puts down our immune system.

Use of antibiotics, cortisone, and synthetic sexual hormones: Antibiotics destroy the bacterian intestinal flora, but not candidas. This allows them to grow without any microorganism to control them. On another side, cortisone puts down the immune system, and the synthetic hormones, among other damages, destroy certain nutrients (like vitamin B6) vital for the immune system's health.

Pregnancy: During this period, our progesterone levels increase, causing the endometrial glands to produce glycogen, which stimulates the growth of candidas.

Continued stress: An excess of cortisol puts down the immune system, increases the glucose levels and destroys the bacterial intestinal flora.

Reduction of digestive secretions: The lack of hydrochloric acid and digestive enzymes prevents us from a correct food digestion, producing intestinal fermentation and putrefaction. This generates substances irritating for the intestinal mucous membrane, favoring the intestinal flora's imbalance and the candidas growth.

Lack of nutrients: We need a great quantity of nutrients, necessary to maintain a healthy immune system, to regulate hormones, to maintain a healthy production of digestive secretions, and to regulate glucose, all factors of vital importance to control candidas. When we suffer undernourishment, candidas have more opportunities to grow.

SYMPTOMS

Candidiasis symptoms are many and very different. It is very important to know why candidiasis can produce those symptoms in order to understand this imbalance. There is a lot of people with candidiasis who haven't been diagnosed and, however, they are treated as hypochondriacs, depressed and/or anxious. Unfortunately, these people are taking Prozac, Seroxat or anxiolytics, instead of following a treatment for candidiasis. Part of this is usually because candidiasis is only related to its own located symptoms caused by the infection. For example, generally with vaginal candidiasis we can only see symptoms located in the vagina; with an oral candidiasis, we pay attention only to the symptoms on our mouth... and treatments are local. However, candidiasis must be analyzed as a whole set, seeing more than just its located manifestation.

A very important point, normally ignored when diagnosing and treating candidiasis, is its intestinal origen, even when we talk about a vaginal candidiasis.

When candidiasis proliferates in the bowel, it can change its anatomy and its physiology. This means that it can stop being a yeast and become a micotic mycelium. It is known that candidas are dimorphic organisms, and they can exist in both forms. In its yeast form, it produces rhizoids (or very long roots) which are highly invasive and can penetrate the mucous membrane. This can cause an excessive permeability of the bowel mucous membrane, allowing the entrance into the blood to substances (toxines, poorly digested proteins, etc) which can act as antigens and seriously alter the immune system. On another hand, an excessive bowel permeability can also deteriorate the cell nutritional receivers, favouring a bad absorption and resulting in undernourishment.
It is known that candidas, in its micotic form, can produce 79 toxic products, among them the most usual

is acetaldehyde.   Sherry Roger, doctor and expert in environmental related diseases, has plenty of published material, absolutely unique and innovative, about acetaldehyde.   Some of the conclusions reached by her and other researchers about the negative effects of this chemical product are:

It favours the production of vasoactive substances, such as adrenaline, causing symptoms like nervousness, panic, fear, tachycardia and hot flushes.
It interferes with the acetylcholine receivers, important for memory and nervous system.
It produces histamine, and with it the swelling of different body parts.
It blocks metabolic enzymes, which can lead to a blockage in the formation of neurotransmitters, to put an example.
It destroys vitamin B6, which is important for mucous membrane protection, immune system strengthening, hormonal system balance, and production of hydrochloric acid and digestive enzymes.
It depresses the immune system.
It destroys the swallowing system and cysteine, essential for body detoxification.
It reacts with dopamine, which can cause depression, insomnia and inability to respond to stress.

On another side, Candidas get into the cell hormonal receivers, getting in competition with the hormones, and they can also create receivers of our own hormones on their surfaces.   This can cause a blockage and imbalance of the hormonal system, and endless problems, with premenstrual, infertility and endometriosis symptoms, among others.

Some yeast like Krusei Candida and Parapsilosis produce thiaminase (an enzyme) which destroys vitamin B1. The lack of this vitamin can produce symptoms like irritability, muscular pain, lack of concentration, stomachache, constipation and tachycardia.

It also prevents the change of vitamin B6 to its active form, piridoxal-5-phosphate. This can cause symptoms like fluid retention, lack of energy, and very dry skin.

Due to the level of toxicity found on Candidiasis patients, the liver must filter a great quantity of chemical products. In order for this to happen, the two desintoxication phases of this organ, phase 1 and 2, require nutrients like zinc, selenium, copper, magnesium, vitamins B and C, glutathione, sulphur, glycine and essential fatty acids, which due to a bad bowel absorption, maybe they aren't found in the correct quantity needed for the desintoxication process. This desintoxication process can aggravate the patient's condition with chronic candidiasis whenever he is in the presence of perfumes, smoke or other chemical inhalants.

The most commong symptoms in chronic
patients are:

- Fatigue
- General discomfort
- Headaches
- Abdominal distension
- Diarrheas and/or constipation
- Indigestion
- Heartburn
- Desire to eat carbohydrates (sweets, pasta, bread, etc).
- Depression
- Dizziness
- Feeling of hangover in the morning
- Pain in joints and muscles
- Vaginal discomfort (itching, irritation, wounds, etc)
- Fluid retention
- Insomnia
- Chronic infections
- Allergies
- Anal itching
- Aphonia
- Nasal congestion
- Suffocation
- Nail problems
- Eye and ear discomfort

The diseases and imbalances related to chronic
candidiasis are:

- Crohn's disease
- Colitis
- Irritable bowel syndrome
- Rheumatoid arthritis

- Lupus
- Asthma
- Psoriasis and Eczema
- Sinusitis
- Multiple sclerosis
- Fibromyalgia
- Chronic fatigue syndrome
- Hypothyroidism
- Hypoglycemia
- Depression and anxiety states
- Anemia

Therefore, the matter of Candidiasis is not only limited to a unique located symptomatology.

DIAGNOSIS

Clinical tests don't guarantee a reliable diagnose for a chronic bowel candidiasis. For example, most candidas cells get stuck to the bowel mucous walls, making it difficult to be seen in a stool test. And, in some cases, many of these cells die while the specimen is transported or while we wait for the analyzing.

It's important not to discard the disease, only because the lab tests turn out to be negative. It's better to base the diagnose on a detailed evaluation of the patient: symptoms, clinical history, analysis of his diet...

In the U.S.A. many doctors and therapists

consider that the clinical protocol for candidiasis presents so little risk and cost (mainly the diet), that it should be considered for any chronic disease.

After all we have exposed, I think it is necessary that all people affected with fibromyalgia do a candidas test.

With this chapter, I only pretend to get to you some information about a disease which often goes along with fibromyalgia.

You must get yourselves in a good specialist's hands, never following a treatment on your own.

This is a very serious disease and, if you suffer with candidas without treatment, you won't be able to improve your fibromyalgia symptoms.

DIET

BREAKFAST

Is very important to take a glass of oatmeal, rice, quinoa, millet. Each person must value which one makes him fill better, and choose it according to his blood group.

You can eat toasts and cookies, sugar free and made of spelt, oatmeal, millet, rice.

We will take now:
2 pills of spirulina + 2 pills of magnesium + 1 pill of vitamin C. We must always make sure these pills make us feel good.

MID-MORNING

In order to avoid the creation of intolerance by our body, we must eat something different each day:
Spelt toast + vegetal pâté.
Rye toast + ham
Bread without yeast + tuna
These are examples of what we can eat by mid-morning, each one can prepare what he prefers always following the recommended guidelines.

You can take coffee or tea sometimes, but better horsetail or three years tea, WITHOUT SUGAR, sweetened with stevia or a bit of rice molasses, agave or syrup.

MID-AFTERNOON

It can be like mid-morning, it all depends on how hungry you are, you can also consider flavoured rice waffles. If we want to loose weight, rice waffles are a good choice.

MONDAY

LUNCH

A plate of legumes with algae
Fish

Salad with lettuce, onion, olives, etc.

DINNER

Chicken soup with rice or spelt pasta
Mere with vegetables

TUESDAY

LUNCH

Boiled green beans or another vegetable.
We can add to it a bit of potatoe or yucca
Fish with grilled vegetables

DINNER

Boiled spinach with a bit of potato or yucca
Vegetable soy burger or homemade burger

WEDNESDAY

LUNCH

Rice pasta with broccoli and onion with a can of
tuna
Salad

DINNER

Chicken stew with vegetables

THURSDAY

LUNCH

Mashed zucchini with onion and a bit of potato
or yucca
Baked chicken

DINNER

Scrambled eggs with young garlic and shrimp

FRIDAY

LUNCH

Fish soup with rice or spelt noodles

Fish
Salad

DINNER

Boiled mixed vegetables
Pork loin battered without egg

SATURDAY

LUNCH

We have several options:
Chicken broth with spelt or rice noodles + fish or white meat
Or pasta with broccoli and onion with meat or tuna

DINNER

Free always respecting the rules

SUNDAY

LUNCH

Paella with meat or fish or Baked rice, always using brown rice
Assorted vegetables or salad
Any dessert without much sugar
Oatmeal, custard, chocolate without milk, homemade
biscuit. It's the only day we can allow ourselves to forget a bit about our diet.

DINNER

Boiled mixed vegetables
Fish
We can eat rice waffles during our meals, oil intake is only restricted if we wish to loose weight.
We must always control that the food we are taking makes us feel good, and we must avoid food with yeast, sugar, dairy products, food that

provokes us intolerance or allergy.
Avoid carrots, fermented foods, vinegar.
Always use yucca, better than potato.

THE DIET

BASIC RECOMMENDATIONS

Mainly, we must follow the recommended diet, according to our blood group, to the letter.   We must have a great willpower to follow it exactly, without falling into the temptation of eating something not beneficial for our blood group, since doing otherwise, the sacrifice we have done(it's a sacrifice at first, even though we enjoy it afterwards) will be of no use and our body will respond with contractures and fatigue.

Besides respecting our form of nutrition according to our blood group, it is very important to follow Dr. Olga Cuevas advise indicated later on, at the end of the food planning for each group.

In second place, it is important to accompany the diet with a physiotherapy to act upon the contractures (the physiotherapist will know how to act upon them without aggravating the problem)

In third place, in long lasting cases, which are affected psychologically, we will also need the support of a psychologist expert in fibromyalgia.

TIME OF RESPONSE

The time of response will be different for each person depending on the years he has suffered the disease and how affected is his body.

Our daughter Marta started to notice the results on the first week.

The first thing she noticed was that she could sleep all night long without waking up and without the need to take any sleeping pills.

Little by little, the pain and the fatigue started to go away. In three weeks, she was a new person, but I have to point out that Marta has been very strict and she has learned how to save her energy on strategic days, for example, when there is an important climate change, wind, cold, etc.

Another thing she has had to learn is not to be ashamed when she eats with her friends, at home or going out, she must only take what she knows is not going to harm her, and she has also taught her friends how to respect her.

VARIOUS SYMPTOMS

There are various symptoms that can appear the first days after beginning a diet.

We must take into consideration that during the

healing process, we can have certain physical symptoms due to abstinence. It is important to know which ones they are, just so we don't confuse them with symptoms of the disease.

Symptoms of a body doing a clean-up can be:

- General fatigue
- Aches and pains
- Fever, chills, cough.
- Abnormal sweating and frequent urination.
- Unusual suppurations and body odors.
- Diarrhea or constipation
- Temporary decrease of sexual desire and vitality.
- Temporary halt of menstrual period.
- Irritable mood.
- Other temporary minor symptoms: Restless sleep, non important hair loss, sensation of cold.

Each person can have some of these symptoms, and the better his general health is, the less symptoms are likely to appear. Also, the symptoms are normally only temporary, and they last only a few hours or a few days.

There are cases of severe liver and kidney intoxication, in which the symptoms of abstination can last up to forty days (just like it happens with drug addiction and its following withdrawal reaction).

Implication by the medical specialists.

NOTE FROM THE AUTHORS:

Very important: Every follow-up process of a diet must be controlled by a medical professional, considering that besides the different symptoms of fibromyalgia suffered by the patient, there can also be bone or muscle injuries which have to be controlled and treated, without abandoning the diet and following all concepts indicated in this book for this purpose.

NUTRITION

We prefer to say that it is not a diet, but a way of eating to last a lifetime, and once you get used to it, it's no big deal. In a few months, your shopping habits will have changed, and they will seem quite normal.

Each blood group has a type of food to combine together, to obtain a healthy, well-balanced and natural diet, and most of all, to contain all the basic nutrients for a good health.

If a type of food, being beneficial, doesn't make us feel good, it must be replaced by another one which gives us the same benefits.

This way of nutrition is based on three foundations:

- Choice of food according to our blood group.
- Nutrition advise from Dr. Olga Cuevas explained later on.
- Mediterranean diet and two year period of work testing and improving on patients affected by fibromyalgia.

The doctor explains to us the chemical reaction produced between our blood and the food we eat:

"This reaction is part of our genetic inheritance. We know it is due to a factor known as lectins, which are proteins found in food and contain properties that may affect our blood".

FRUITS

Since childhood, we are taught to eat fruit right after our meals. Fruit is a vital food for a good health, it prevents from illness, it gives us lots of nutrients needed by our body, and of course it provides us with authentically vital and healthy energy.

But according to some nutritionists, the problem is the moment when we eat fruit, always as a dessert, and accompanied with other food. Most fruits, except bananas, take little time to be digested in our stomach. Due to that reason, we must eat fruit alone, with an empty stomach, by the middle of the morning or afternoon, never together with any other food.

This way, all their nutrients and vitamins will be absorbed correctly by our body, and they won't produce a sensation of bloating, burning or flatulence when entering in contact with other food and fermenting in our stomach.

CALCIUM

According to Dr. Olga Cuevas Fernandez, in the book "Balance through Nutrition", calcium is the most abundant mineral in our body. Its main function is to help in the construction and maintenance of bones and teeth, along with phosphorous. It also participates in the correct heart and neuromuscular system's function.

In fact, there isn't an agreement among researchers about the quantity of calcium that we need, although there are factors that ease or complicate the intestinal calcium absorption.

SUGAR AND REFINED PRODUCTS

Refined products, specially the sugared ones, don't contain any minerals. These type of products steals calcium from our bones for their neutralization, when the kidneys have reached their limit of disposal of metabolic acids.

They also produce a lack of minerals, mainly magnesium, essential for bone formation. After a considerable sugar intake, there is an increase of calcium disposal through urine.

After some years following a diet low in magnesium and calcium, the body ends up suffering its consecuences.

A calcium shortage is corrected by magnesium intake, and not calcium. Magnesium favors vitamin D absorption, essential to help calcium go throught the intestinal walls (we get vitamin D with sun-bathing or eating blue fish to maintain our liver and kidneys in a good condition).

When we take calcium supplements or eat food enriched with calcium, we should take into consideration that it is of organic or natural origin and not from a synthetic source. Organic- comes from green leaf vegetables, nuts and mostly from algae.

THE OTHER FACE OF DAIRY PRODUCTS
Doctor Olga Cuevas explains:

"Milk is a complete nutrient, by itself it can nourish and cause a baby to grow. Laboratory tests prove that it has proteins, fats, carbohydrates, minerals and vitamins totally appropriate for the infant. For that reason, they have made us believe that if we don't take dairy products, we will loose our teeth, our bones will disintegrate, and our children won't grow up.

Nevertheless, common sense tells us that milk is suitable for infants, and we see in Nature that adult animals don't suck milk from their mothers, and even less from females of other species. Common sense doesn't deceive, milk is to be sucked; and in fact, once milked it starts to spoil very quickly. Men solves it by sterilization with heat. That way it becomes drinkable, but have you asked yourself if it has the same benefits and if it is as easy to digest as the one from the breast?

And, is it the same to suck from your mother as from a cow?"

We get nourishment from what we retain, not from what we eat.

The antigenic character of milk proteins

> The human baby totally retains the caseins from his mother's milk, but he can't do the same with cow's milk caseins, which pass to the small intestine partially digested, due to the neutralizing effect of milk over the stomach acid, needed for its breakdown. This problem gets worse in adults, with age the gastric renin decreases in quantity, this is the first enzyme needed to start the beakdown chain of the casein molecules.
>
> Non hydrolyzed casein (fragmented) is a viscose substance which, in some people, is placed in the lymphatic follicles that surround the intestine, preventing the absorption of other nutrients and promoting the chronic fatigue and other intestinal disorders. In ideal conditions, non digested and non decomposed milk proteins and other food antigens, are retained in the bowel and expelled along with stools. In people with IgA deficiency, proteins like the difficult to digest casein, are totally absorbed in the blood flow and they participate in the development of a number of diseases related to autoimmunity, including rheumatical arthritis, lupus, cancer...

In summary: dairy products have high levels of antigens which "exhaust" the immune system, making us more vulnerable to infection and diseases related with our immune system.

There are lots of problems related to dairy products. Among them are: circulation problems, allergies, immunodepression, juvenile diabetes, otorhinolaryngological diseases, asthma, mucous accumulation, specially in female genital organs and auditory system.

According to the French doctor Gauvin, throat, nose and ear diseases are due to the high intake of yogurt and milk, and doctor Oski, head of the pediatric hospital John Hopkins, assures that many cases of asthma and sinusitis get better or even disappear when dairy products are totally removed from the diet.

All people with health problems should reduce their dairy product intake, but those who have skin or respiratory allergies should eliminate them completely, as well as all industrial food containing casein.

Caseins are present in all dairy products (milk, cheese, yogurt) being more problematic in industrial cheese, due to their higher concentration

ARE DAIRY PRODUCTS A CALCIUM SOURCE

Dairy products are not a good calcium source. Doctor William Ellis affirms that after more than 25000 blood tests, he discovered that the lowest calcium levels were found in people used to taking three, four or five glasses of milk every day.

Milk substitutes

In fact, we can perfectly eat without any type of deficiencies leaving dairy products aside. The need to replace dairy products by others only responds to two reasons: one is our worry about getting calcium; the other one, our psychological attachment to our daily breast-feeding.

About calcium, we should worry more about its loss that about its intake, and include in our diet a good quantity of vegetables (cabbage, broccoli, parsley...) algae, oatmeal milk, rice with algae and sesame.

Excess of proteins

A high intake of proteins increases the kidney disposal of calcium. There is evidence that osteoporosis is less common and less severe in people who eat little meat.

For better bowel absorption of calcium

- Avoid taking antiacids and farmacologic extended treatments with corticoids, etc. They can block the absorption of certain minerals and vitamins. That's why it's better to avoid them if not necessary.
- Avoid industrial food with phosphates as additives (E-442,E-450, and from E-338 to E343), they are found in: Sausages, melted cheese, dairy

creams, canned fruit and carbonated drinks, among others
- Take blue fish and green leaves.
- Avoid carbonated drinks.

ALGAE

They are the oldest vegetables, and their assimilation is excellent.

They are in Nature among the richest products in calcium and iron.   They also have important quantities of vitamins, aminoacids, enzymes, iodine, magnesium, sulphur, chlorine, manganese,...

Being very concentrated, they must not be taken in big quantities.   About 10 grams a day provide us enough minerals and vitamins.

Among algae properties, we can quote:
- Mineralizing
- Metabolic stimulants
- Regulation of kidneys and blood flow
- Help to eliminate fluids
- Alcalinizers

Algae are used as food but also as supplements to reinforce the skeleton, hair and nails; treat cardiovascular problems; loose weight ; lower cholesterol levels; help eliminate tumors; anemia; osteoporosis; hypothyroidism; help in desintoxication process...

People who suffer tachycardia with many palpitations, and those who take iodine or have hyperthyroidism, should control their intake.

Due to their high contents of iodine, people with hypertension or heart problems should use them in small quantities and better toasted to allow part of the iodine to be evaporated.

There are many varieties of algae and each one has its own properties.

Arame
Very rich in iron and calcium, very useful to give elasticity to the cardiovascular system and for anemia.

Iziki
Very rich in calcium and iron, and very useful for osteoporosis.

Nori
They have a big quantity of vitamin A; very rich in proteins and vitamin B12, besides they contain calcium, iron, potassium, vitamin C and vitamins of group B.

Kombu
They are the richest in iodine, they help to eliminate bowel toxics, besides being very remineralizing, due to their high contents of iron. They

are also rich in vitamins of group B and pro vitamin A.

Wakame

They are very rich in calcium and other minerals. They are the richest in vitamins of group B, they activate the circulation and help to balance the nervous system.

Spirulina

The spirulina alga is probably one of the foods on which men have researched the most during the last half century. Perhaps, it is because due to its nutritional qualities it could, by itself, relieve the hunger that devastates the world. It is an alga which contains:

Proteins and aminoacids.
Its content of proteins is, on average, higher than 65% of any other natural food. Only 36 grams of spirulina satisfy the daily requierement of aminoacids needed for an average adult. In fact, spirulina contains all the essential amionacids we know.

Vitamins.
It's the richest food in beta carotene and pro Vitamin A,   it's also   the   most important source of vitamin B12 and it provides with considerable quantities of B1 and B2.

Minerals.
It's the food with the richest content of iron known so far, even twenty times more than

others which are considered as vital sources of this mineral. Ten grams of spirulina, for example, give us the 80% of the recommended daily needs. It also has important concentration of calcium and magnesium, and with the advantage that it contains almost no sodium.

Lipids (fats).
Spirulina contents of fats go between 4 and 7%, very low compared with other sources of proteins. Ten grams of this alga have only 36 calories and practically no cholesterol. Besides, almost all the fats it contains are essential fatty acids of type omega 6.

Carbohydrates .
It contains a very small quantity of sugar. Besides, this food gives fast energy without Overloading the pancreas or developing hypoglycemia.

Gammalinolenic fatty acid (GLA).
It is, along with mother's milk, the only food that contains noticeable quantities of this fatty acid which cooperates in the regulation of all our hormonal network.

** Note: This article about spiruline, comes from the report Algae: Marine Vegetables, from the magazine: Discovery D health, number 66, which tells us about the importance of algae in our nutrition.*

MILLET

Millet is a yan cereal, being one of the most versatile and oldest cereals.

Of all gramineae, it is the most alkalizing; very rich in proteins, minerals (specially magnesium and iron) and Lecitine.

It is very digestive, it benefits the stomach and the spleen-pancreas. Very useful for diabetics. It is a cereal without gluten, which makes it apt for celiacs. It contains silicon, necessary to preserve skin, nails and hair in good conditions.

Millet comes from central Africa, and from there it expanted to China and India. It was one of the first cereals used by mankind. Nowadays, it is used by more than 400 million people around the world, mostly in China, India, North Africa and Europe.

It's a cereal which is used more each day due to its virtues, it tastes good, it's sweet, light and alkalizing. Besides, it is more nutritious, more energetic and richer in mineral salts than the rest of the cereals commonly spread.

It has a high level of proteins and it is, along with oatmeal, the most energetic cereal that we know, as well as rich in iron, calcium, phosphorous, patassium, sodium, magnesium, zinc, manganese, and vitamins A, B and PP.

Its contents of magnesium make it a great calcium fixer.

Its intake is highly positive for bone development and of great benefit for pancreas, spleen, and for people who have diabetes. It helps, enormously, our eye conditions and our stomach problems.

Due to its versatility, it has been traditionally the substitute of rice in almost all countries where it is implanted. And being the sweetest of all cereals, it can be adapted to sweet and to sour dishes.

Concerning fibromyalgia, and according to our own experience, we must tell you that millet has given us a natural way to nourish Marta with food that gives her energy, in the morning, which we had not been able to give her before.

We take millet at home as cereals for breakfast, always using pealed biological seeds, boiled in water and spiced to each person's taste, it may be sweet or salty.

We can also add it to soups or desserts. At the end of the book, we include some recipes with millet, by "Light of Life".

MAGNESIUM

According to Doctor Olga Cuevas Fernandez, magnesium is one of the most important minerals. It is distributed through our entire body and it participates directly in the most important physiological functions: make up and subsequent use of the high energy unions, base for all metabolic reactions, it intervenes in the synthesis of all type of proteins, antibodies, neurotransmitters, enzymes, hormones, collagen,... being of vital importance in the transmission of nervous impulse and in most of the cellular exchanges.

A lack of magnesium produces a great symptomatology:

- Anxious hyper emotionality, nervousness, tired voice, tightness in chest, trembling, headaches, vertigo, and insomnia.

- Itching, tingling, cramps, contractions, excessive fatigue, nail, hair and teeth fragility.

The daily requirements of magnesium are around 350 mg/day, but they increase if we take food very rich in potassium, calcium supplements or with lots of proteins, sugar and refined foods.

Dairy products interfere in their absorption. Diuretics and strong laxatives eliminate magnesium. But the biggest "thief" of magnesium is sugar, because it increases its elimination through urine.

UMEBOSHI

Umeboshi plums are one of the most characteristic products of Japan. Ume plums are submitted to a fermentation process with salt and shiso leaves from one to three years, increasing their contents of citric acid, one of their most important elements for their healthy effects.

Citric acid is used by our body to break down lactic acid (which excess produces fatigue) into carbon dioxide and water.

The acid found in umeboshi neutrilizes the excess of YAN (meat, salt, proteins) while the salt contained in them neutralizes the YIN state originated by the excess of sugar, refined cereals and other food with expansive polarity.

They stimulate the bowels, the liver and the gallbladder, they alkalize the blood and increase our body defenses.

UMEBOSHI PLUMS CAN BE USED FOR:

- Problems caused by lack of liver energy.
- To segregate saliva and prepare digestion.
- As alkalizer.
- For digestive hepatic problems.
- To metabolize sugar excess.
- To eliminate radioactivity.
- To stop growth of bacteria.

- As tranquilizer for stress.
- For intestinal disorders (diarrhea ,constipation).
- To help in calcium absorption.
- To stop fatigue.
- To delay aging process.
- They are useful with food poisoning.
- To help with car sickness, ship dizziness, etc.

Important: Due to its contents of salt, we should not abuse if we have high blood pressure or an excess of YAM.

KUZU

Kuzu is a starch taken out, through a long traditional process, from volcanic roots which sometimes go as much as two meters deep. These roots are ground and washed repeatedly with pure mountain water and air dried during ninety days.

It comes from China and during two millenniums it has been part of its culture. Tea from its roots was described in Chinese medicine as antipyretic, antidiarrhea, sweat producing and anti vomit.

Even though kuzu has a very old usage, it has only been studied by scientists during the last three decades.

In these studies, they have proved its effectiveness on the cardiovascular and cardiocerebral systems, with application on angina pectoris, migraines and headaches, hypertension and sudden deafness.

KUZU CAN BE USED AT HOME:

- Helping to discharge the liver, joint pains, hepatitis, cirrhosis, alcoholism...
- Regenerating intestinal flora. Neutralizing toxic excess in the bowels.
- For flu with painful I.G. points.
- For allergies with rhinitis.
- To reduce inflammation of bowel: diarrhea,colitis, typhus, crown, salmonella.
- For lung problems with their origin in weakness of the large intestine, asthma, bronchitis.
- To reduce fever.
- In infectious process.
- In skin problems.
- In lack of memory or analysis capacity: depression, Alzheimer.

HOW TO USE UMEBOSHI AND KUZU IN FIBROMYALGIA.

In our case, we have used these two foods/medicines to recover Marta's intestinal flora.

Marta used to suffer with morning diarrhea which supposed a big ordeal in her everyday life, mostly at the moment of leaving the home in the morning.

We decided to use these foods, advised by a

naturalist physician, and just a few days later, she started feeling better, and the discomfort improved. She still takes them at night.

The way to prepare it is as follows:

In a small glass of water, we add a teaspoon of kuzu, stir it and heat it in a pot during three minutes until it thickens, we remove it from the heat and add a bit of umeboshi, let it cool down and take it while it is still warm.

As a personal opinion, we believe it's very important for our body to take these foods/medicines. We strongly recommend them.

SUGAR

According to doctor Olga Cuevas Fernandez, sugar (and other sweeteners) is one of the worst foods for our body, specially due to our abuse of it.

In the refinement process, we not only take all the fiber away from beets or sugar canes, but also their minerals, vitamins and oligoelements.

The nutrients of beet or cane saccharose are the tools it needs to be metabolized. The body must use its wit to pull out the nutrients lost by refinement, from other foods or from its own tissues, creating a vitamin deficiency, especially of group B, a mineral deficiency (mostly magnesium) and an oligoelements deficiency.

Sugar and Bones

After the intake of a considerable quantity of sugar, there is an increase of urinary calcium disposal.

When sugar metabolizes, it produces acid wastes and for their neutralization, calcium comes out of the bones. Bones get weak and, with the time, this takes us to the so feared osteoporosis.

Sugar and Lipids (Fats)

When we take sugar we introduce in our stomach enormous quantities of caloric material in excess, which will be stored as body fat.

With the excess of sweets, we won't only see our weight go up, but also our cholesterol and other fats in our blood, which will increase and bring to us cardiovascular diseases.

Besides our direct use of refined sugar and sweeteners, most industries use them to elaborate their products. We find it in candies, soft drinks, pastries, sandwich bread, prepared sauces, breakfast cereals, canned food, sausages, etc. Many people take excessive quantities of sugar without even knowing it.

* Doctor Olga Cuevas Fernandez is licensed in Chemical Science by the University of Salamanca and doctor in Biochemistry by the University Complutense of Madrid.   She has done a lot of work in scientific research, published in international prestige magazines, in the department of chemical enzyme and medical chemistry in the National Center of Organic Chemistry of the Superior Institute of Scientific Investigations of Madrid, and research works with natural products in the Sussex University (UK). She is a specialist in Nutrition and Health by the Politechnical University of Madrid.

We want to thank her for the knowledge we have found in her book "Balance through Nutrition" which has contributed in our daughter's recovery.

BOWEL HYPERSENSITIVITY

BOWEL HYPERSENSITIVITY

According to Doctor Olga Cuevas, some autoimmune diseases like rheumatoid arthritis, lupus, thyroid and fibromyalgia can be a consecuence of abowel hyperpermeability.

The bowel walls are porous in order to allow the passage of nutrients into the blood; at the same time, the intestinal mucous membrane acts as a brake to stop the entrance in our body to food that hasn't been totally digested, to toxics or to harmful microorganisms.

The bowel barrier is not perfect, and it's easy for some intruders to "go in", which doesn't suppose a problem for most individuals. The real problems begins when the bowel walls swell and become hyperpermeable. That is to say, this happens to people who, due to genetic reasons, have their bowel wall thinner than normal, or for different reasons they get them swollen during the assimilation process, causing not only nutrients but also waste substances and food toxics to go through the bowel walls.

These get to the liver and the kidneys for their elimination, but being flooded, the immune system appears, who considers them enemies, and declares them a war. This implies a vitamin wear for the body, and toxic substances are produced which can be accumulated in different parts of the body, causing injuries at different levels (in bones, in muscles, neuromuscular).

Swelling may happen due to different reasons, among them are:

- Abnormal intestinal flora produced mostly by abuse of antibiotics, which destroy good bacterian flora and allow the development of yeasts and harmful fungi.
- The abuse of animal products and the intake of little fiber, which favour the development of coli bacteria, which cause putrefaction in detriment of the beneficial acidophilus.
- Substances that irritate the digestive tract, like alcohol, caffeine, additives, spices, sugar...
- Food intolerance, for example, milk, gluten, or other foods, which can be detected through blood tests.
- The abuse of fermented foods, bread, cheese, alcohol, pickles...
- Water intake or other foods contaminated by microorganisms.
- Treatment with steroids and non steroid antiinflamatories, including aspirin. This is the most important cause of bowel hyperpermeability. These medicines swell the bowel walls and cause the widening of spaces between cells.
- Intake of non allowed food according to our blood group.

Consequences of bowel swelling and hyperpermeability

- When the bowel gets swollen, it doesn't absorb like it should, and it can produce gas, swelling, abdominal pain, indigestion, constipation and diarrhea.
- The proteins being transported can result injured and cause a nutrient deficiency, which can also lead to any other symptoms, this happens with magnesium deficiency, which leads to muscular spasms or with copper deficiency, which leads to high cholesterol levels.
- Toxin leakage through the bowel walls, overloads the liver and it can cause sensitivity to chemical products and to new foods.
- Bowel bacteria and fungi acquire the capacity to move to other body parts causing injuries.

THE IMPORTANCE OF CARBOHYDRATES FOR THE PRODUCTION OF SEROTONINA.

Some pharmaceutical products, like antidepressants or anxiolytics, cause a great addiction. But besides, they produce severe alterations and liver problems.

At first, when we take them, we have a feeling of relief, but when we spend some time taking them, apart from a high level of addiction, they cause many physical and mental problems.

Doctor Olga Cuevas explains what we must do to produce serotonina by ourselves. This will enable patients who are taking antidepressants to stop taking them quickly.

With enough intake of carbohydrates in our diet, the liver not only maintains a normal level of glucose in blood, but it can store a good quantity of glycogen, and reduce to the minimum the demolition speed of proteins and the protein oxidation.

The quantity of carbohydrates in our diet regulates the demolition speed of fats and proteins.

A diet low in carbohydrates can cause an acetone attack, hypoglycemic states, low blood sugar and *depression*.

If the quantity of carbohydrates in our diet is very low, the blood-brain barrier, customs entrance to the brain, has no choice but restrict the entrance of aminoacids, *especially tryptophan*, due to the few carbohydrates provided.

When the entrance of the aminoacid tryptophan into the brain is limited, we can't produce the neurotransmitter serotonina.

This causes in us states of irritability, anguish, increase of sensitivity to pain, and depression.

In summary, we must eat more carbohydrates,

pasta, bread, but all of spelt and rice, and better if they are whole grain.

THE ACID/ALKALINE BALANCE

We form in our metabolism, and in a natural way, acid compounds which are latter eliminated or neutralized: some of them turn into carbon dioxide and water, and are expelled through the lungs, skin and kidneys; others are used by the stomach in the form of hydrochloric acid; others are neutralized and expelled as salts through the kidneys; and others are neutralized by the minerals from the alkaline foods that stay in our metabolism.

The acid/alkaline balance is measured by the blood pH, the pH scale goes from 0 to 14, and the pH 7 is neutral (like water's), less than 7 is acid and more than 7 is alkaline or basic.

The blood pH must stay constant to allow the many metabolic functions that make our life possible. For this, our body must counteract the inclination to acidity or alkalinity that generates each vital process.

Causes of acidosis
- Inability for the kidney to get rid of acids.
- Inability for the lungs to get rid of carbon dioxide.
- Liver alterations.
- Metabolic alterations, excessive production of acids.
- Diet with too many acids that are not metabolized.

- Diarrhea.
- Diet with predominance of acidifying food.
- Stress.
- Hard work.
- Excessive sun exposure.
- Intestinal fermentations.
- Fasting and ketogenic diets (based on meat of fat).

Causes of alkalosis

They are not very common, only:
- After an episode of continued vomiting when reducing the quantity of gastric acid.
- Due to an excess of hyperventilation.
- As a consequence to having taken a high dose of antiacids.

Possible symptoms of acidosis
- Chronic lack of energy, ease to fatigue and cold, swollen and sensitive gums, dental cavities, dull hair, dry skin, weak nails, cramps, muscle spasms, joint problems, ease to get infections, ease for distress, pain when pressing muscles, ease for depression.

ACID/ALKALINE FOODS

Classification

-Alkaline:
- Rich in mineral salts: Algae, vegetables, fruits, natural wine, tea, bananas, chestnuts, almonds, leafy vegetables, gomasio and salt.

-Neutral:
- There are foods that due to their protein content are acidifying, and due to their mineral salts content are alkalizing. These are the neutral foods: Pasteurized milk, milk serum, tofu, whole grain cereals, and cheese.

-Acidifying:
- Alcohol, sugar, fats and oils, raw tomatoes, fatty fruits, white flour, legumes, refined cereals, fish, poultry, meats and eggs.
- Fruits contain acids that are completely metabolized into energy by vital people when the weather is hot.
- On the contrary, little vital people, little resistant to cold, who get tired easily, have problems to metabolize and eliminate these acids, getting some of the symptoms of acidification: Very sensible respiratory mucous membranes, painful sensation on teeth, cold, nervousness, insomnia, fatigue about an hour after eating fruit, cramps and spasms.
- In my own experience, fruit produces these symptoms to me, especially cold, swelling and fatigue. All people are not the same and each must listen to his own body, it is the best way to follow a diet which allow us to be healthy and strong.

Our Proposal

Based on doctors D'Adamo/Catherine Whitney's recommendations, we have tried to elaborate some diets associated to our eating culture and with products that are easy to find in most supermarkets and natural food stores, and for this reason we have included : fish, fruits, grains, legumes and meat, maintaining a balance.

Our body cannot abuse of any type of food, a normally healthy food, may be harmful taken in excess.

ALLERGIES AND OTHER DISEASES
In case of a food allergy, we must remove it immediately and substitute it by another one which is beneficial or neutral, with nutritive properties, and as similar as possible.

Other diseases: In case of high sugar levels, cholesterol, etc. we will need a personal diet for each case.

BENEFICIAL, NEUTRAL AND HARMFUL FOODS
Foods are classified as beneficial when our blood is compatible with its nutritive substances. This food acts as a medicine for our body.

Neutral when it gives us nourishment without complications or benefits.

Harmful when they must not be taken under any circumstances, because taking harmful substances for the body will cause that our liver works harder than it should, and it will weaken the rest of the organs, making us feel bad, having contractures and fatigue. This food acts like a poison.

When preparing a diet, it is important taking into consideration the acid/alkaline balance of foods.

The 80% of the diet should be of alkaline foods. Alkaline foods are: Fruits, vegetables, algae, some nuts and sesame.

Neutral foods are:
Soy, brown rice and whole grain spelt flower.

Acid foods are:
Meat, fish, eggs and milk.

RECOMMENDATIONS:
Take magnesium in pills (do not exceed the daily recommended quantity, a pill with 65 mg of magnesium ion would be almost enough to cover the daily need of a person), besides being very alkaline, it is a wonderful food for the muscles.

If we take calcium supplements we must make sure they are of organic origin (algae, shark cartilage, etc), this will allow us a good calcium assimilation.

If the calcium is of animal or synthetic origin, our body will not be able to assimilate it, producing the opposite effect to the one we want.

By mid-morning we can eat a sandwich (50gr) of spelt bread with ham, sheep's cheese or turkey.

CEREALS AS SOURCE OF LIFE

Spelt

- There are in the market all kinds of spelt products (spelt is a primitive wheat, ecological and not changed genetically, which is appropriate for all types of blood groups).

- We can find sugar-free cookies, pizza bases, macaroni, spaghetti, bread and flour.

- All products derived from wheat (bread, pastries, flours, cookies, etc.) must be replaced by spelt wheat.

Rice

- In the rice refinement process, it looses a big part of its vitamins and suffers a deficiency of vitamin B. That is why we recommend brown rice.

- We can look for pre-cooked brown rice in dietary stores.

Oatmeal

- Known as one of the most energetic and complete cereals, oatmeal has been the nutritional base for some strong nations like Scottish, Irish and some Asian civilizations. Besides, it has the property of warming up the body, which makes it very appropriate for places with cold climate. In its composition we can find a great concentration of proteins: Of the eight essential aminoacids for our life, oatmeal has six. It is the cereal with the biggest quantity of them.

- Oatmeal is also in first place of its species in quantity of lipids: even though it is the most complete in vegetable fats cereal, it doesn't make us fat. In its contents of vitamins and minerals, we find: vitamins B1, B2, E and D, niacin, copper, and zinc. Taking into consideration vitamins like B3 or niacin and its richness in phosphorous, it is clear that oatmeal is very beneficial for our brain activity. It's also an important source of carbohydrates of slow absorption, which give us energy long after their intake.

- Finally, and to complete the long list of inherent components of this powerful cereal, we must point out its contents of fiber, important for digestion, cholesterol and diabetes. All these virtues make oatmeal a food without comparison when we consider quality and quantity of beneficial properties.

- Apart from its energetic properties, it is good for the heart, it reduces cholesterol, it desintoxicates the blood and it prevents from thrombosis, heart attacks and arteriosclerosis.

- It is digestive, it protects the intestinal wall, it doesn't make us fat, it prevents the formation of dental cavities, and it remineralizes the bones. It's important for the nervous system's good functioning, and it helps to ease depression. It stimulates mother's milk, it favours physical and intellectual growth in children, and of course, it helps teeth to grow.

This article comes from the Sunday edition of "El Periodico" 14-11-04 "Vida Sana" signed by U.M.

Oatmeal Milk
- For groups A, B and AB, it is almost essential taking oatmeal milk in the morning and in the afternoon. This gives us organic calcium of easy assimilation as well as magnesium and other minerals.

- For group O, we advise to alternate almond powdered milk without sugar or fructose, and rice milk enriched with organic calcium and magnesium coming from algae.

Diet Samples. Common to all blood group

DIET SAMPLE FOR ALL BLOOD GROUPS

BREAKFAST
- One glass of vegetable milk (oatmeal, millet, almond, soy)
- Or a cream of cereals, of the ones mentioned before.
- Or a three years tea
- Toast of any whole grain cereal (spelt flour, rye) WITHOUT YEAST.
- Or breakfast cereals of oatmeal, millet, quinoa or spelt.

Two pills of spirulina and two pills of magnesium.

MID-MORNING OR MID-AFTERNOON
- Soy yogurt, if you don't have soy intolerance.

- Or one glass of vegetable drink or a cookie or spelt toast with some protein.

MONDAY

LUNCH

Chicken broth with legumes, with brown rice and vegetables, or with rice pasta.
White fish.
An infusion.

DINNER
Vegetables and algae soup.
Vegetable hamburger.
Meals can be accompanied by rice wafers

TUESDAY

LUNCH
Mashed zucchini and onion with oil.
Turkey breast.

DINNER
Vegetables cooked in a bit of oil.
Fish

WEDNESDAY

LUNCH
Rice,spelt or alga macaroni, whole grain if possible
Broccoli and onion cooked with oil.
We can add some tuna in olive oil.

DINNER
Boiled cabbage with oil.
Baked chicken.

THURSDAY

LUNCH
Baked brown rice.
Fry red pepper and onion, add rice with
some chicken or turkey and bake.

DINNER
Spinach with legumes,very little legumes.
Blue or white fish.

FRIDAY

LUNCH

Fish broth with rice or spelt pasta.
Blue or white fish with vegetables.

DINNER

Egg with vegetables.

SATURDAY

LUNCH

Boiled green beans, potato (or better yucca) and onion.
Turkey breast.

DINNER

We can eat what we want, always respecting our blood group and its rules.

SUNDAY

LUNCH

Being a family day, we can eat the same as other members of the family, but avoiding harmful foods.

DINNER

Vegetables
Fish

COMMENTS:

As dessert, we can eat cookies made of rice, spelt or any of the described cereals, avoid the ones with sugar or any components that are harmful for our body.

A very healthy food we can add to our diet is MILLET. It will give us strength. We can eat it as a cereal for breakfast, or in soups.

We can also prepare delicious desserts at home with whole grain flours of spelt, rice, rye, millet. As sweetener, we can use molasses (without abusing) and as excipient to make the dough rise, Royal baking powder (or any other brand), but never baker's yeast.

Drink water on meals. If we have to go out, one glass of wine is allowed.

Never beer or other alcoholic drinks.

If we like salads, we can eat them to our taste. But always paying attention to how it makes us feel afterwards, if we sleep well at night...

We can use salt on our food.

Avoid vinegar.

We can use other cereals in our lunch or dinner like quinoa or buckwheat.

If we tolerate soy, we can have a soy yogurt by mid-morning or mid-afternoon.

The most important part of this diet is learning to

adapt it to our eating habits and make it as natural and easy as possible, it will be the best way of having a good health and enjoying life. And remember BE HAPPY.

BLOOD GROUP

GROUP "O" See
diet on page 95

They are descendants of the first inhabitants of the earth, who were hunters-gatherers, and whose diet was based on fish and fruits, they can eat different types of meat, but always in a balanced way.   They also need regular and intense physical activity, in order to maintain a general balance, physical and mental.

VERY HARMFUL FOOD (NEVER EAT IT)

Wheat, cauliflower, lentils, potatoes, strawberries, oranges, bananas, coffee, corn, cow or goat milk.

COMMENTS

- Sugar is very harmful, its intake must be restricted. It must be replaced by syrup or molasses, with moderation.
- Tuna must be taken fresh or canned in olive oil.
- Olive oil must be taken in moderation.
- Replace bread on meals by brown rice wafers, or any other variety of wafers. Or by 25 gr. of spelt bread.

RECOMMENDED FOODS FOR GROUP "O"

Flours and pasta

☺ Group "O" may combine spelt flour or pasta with barley or rye flour, or with quinoa, kamut or buckwheat products.

☹ Not advisable the intake of wheat and wheat pasta.

Dairy products

😐 They must restrict their intake. They can tolerate mozzarella, goat or sheep cheese and soy.

Nuts and seeds

☺ They can be a good source of vegetal protein. Advisable: walnuts, pumpkin seeds, almonds, hazelnuts, chestnuts, sunflower seeds or sesame seeds.

☹ Not advisable: Peanuts and pistachios.

Legumes

😐 They must be taken with moderation together with vegetables. Advisable: pinto beans, facepiece beans, green beans, kidney beans, peas, garbanzo beans, lima beans and soy germ.

☹ Lentils are not advisable.

Meat

☺ People of group "O" tolerate meat very well, but it must be eaten with moderation. Advisable: Lamb, turkey, chicken, beef, rabbit, quail, hen or duck.

Fish

☺Sea products are the most appropriate in the diet for Group "O". Advisable: herring, cod, mackerel, sole, hake, perch, swordfish, salmon, sardine, trout, anchovy, sea bream, squid, sea snail, prawns, lobster, shrimp, mussels, mere, oysters and pike.

Vegetables

☺There are lots of vegetables available for this group, for example: chards, garlic, artichokes, sweet potatoes, broccoli, cabbage, pumpkin, onion, kale, endive, parsnip, beets, lettuce, turnip, parsley, red bell pepper, leeks, radish, green olives, celery, water cress, asparagus, lima beans, mushrooms, carrots or zucchini.

☹ Not advisable: potatoes and cauliflower.

Fruits

☺There are lots of tasty fruits available in the diet for type "O", for example: black, green or red plums, dry figs, pineapple, persimmon, cherries, apricots, pomegranate, kiwi, lemon, mango, apple, melon, papaya, pear, watermelon and grapes.

☹ Not advisable: oranges, strawberries and bananas.

Drinks

☺There are few drinks acceptable for Group "O", for example: Seltz water, mineral water, beer, green tea, red wine and white wine.

☹ But not advisable: coffee, soda, cola, destilled liquors and black tea.

In our case, this diet done during eight weeks, followed by the letter, has given us great results.

After the eight weeks, if you want more variety in your diet, there are three factors to take into consideration:

1st.-See food recommendations explained before, and the list of foods indicated for each group on their corresponding chapter.

2nd.- Take into consideration some of the advise concerning foods to be avoided or reduced from Doctor Olga Cuevas:

- Fried food, eggs, asparagus, eggplant, spinach, beets, and peppers.
- Red meats, animal fat, sausages, dairy products (milk, cheese, yogurt, butter)
- Margarine.
- Sugar, honey, syrups and other sweeteners (to sweeten we can use a small quantity of molasses of rice or barley)
- All food that contains chemical products, dyes, pesticides or all products of chemical cultivation.
- Refined food and cereals and white flour.
- Strong spices, seasonings and exciting drinks.

3rd.-Follow a Mediterranean diet, in which fish prevails over meat, rich in fruit and with variety of vegetables, without forgetting carbohydrates. (pre-cooked brown rice, whole grain spelt wheat)

In our diet, we should try to include, twice a week, rice and spelt pasta.

We must consider salads very important, trying to eat them in all our meals, we recommend to include in them: lettuce, onion and carrots.

LIST OF FOODS FOR GROUP "O"

Grains and Pasta
- Beneficial
  - None.
- Neutral
  - Rice, barley, rye, spelt, buckwheat.
- Not advisable
  - Couscous, wheat pasta, oatmeal, wheat flour.

Bread
- Beneficial
  - Essene bread, Ezekiel bread.
- Neutral
  - Rice biscuit, rye bread, spelt bread, soy bread, millet bread.
- Not advisable
  - Wheat bread, multicereal bread, corn bread, English bread.

Cereals
- Beneficial
  - None
- Neutral
  - Rice, barley, spelt, millet, buckwheat.
- Non advisable
  - Assorted cereals, wheat, starch, wheat germ, oatmeal, corn.

Nuts
- Beneficial
  - Walnut, pumpkin seeds.
- Neutral
  - Sesame seeds, hazelnuts, almonds, chestnuts, sunflower seeds.
- Not advisable
  - Peanuts, pistachios

Meats
- Beneficial
  - Bull, deer, ram, lamb, liver, beef.
- Neutral
  - Quail, rabbit, pheasant, hen, duck, turkey, partridge, chicken.
- Not advisable
  - Pork, goose, bacon.

Fish and seafood
- Beneficial
  - Herring, cod, mackerel, sturgeon, sole, pike, hake, perch, swordfish, salmon, trout.
- Neutral
  - Pout, clams, anchovies, eel, sea bream, squid, crab, sea snails, carp, cazon, prawns, lobster, shrimp, sole, mussels, mere, oysters.

- Not advisable
  - Smoked herring, caviar, barracuda, octopus, smoked salmon, scallops.

Dairy products
  - Beneficial
    - None
  - Neutral
    - Butter, soy milk, goat cheese, sheep cheese, soy cheese, fresh cheese, mozzarella.
  - Not advisable
    - Brie, Camembert, Cottage, Emmenthal, skimmed cheese, ice cream, Gruyere, Kefir, whole milk, skimmed milk, goat milk, Parmesan, Edam , Gouda, Swiss cheese, Roquefort, yogurt.

Drinks
  - Beneficial
    - Seltz water, mineral water.
  - Neutral
    - Beer, green tea, white and red wine
  - Not advisable
    - Coffee, soda, cola, destilled liquors, black tea

Juices and Liquids
  - Beneficial
    - Pineapple juice, plum juice, cherry juice
  - Neutral
    - Juices made of celery, blueberries, cucumber, apricot, tomatoes, grape, carrot.
  - Not advisable
    - Apple cider, cabbage juice, apple juice.

Fruits
  - Beneficial
    - Plums, figs, prunes

- Neutral
    - Pineapple, cherries, dates, raspberries,
      pomegranate, kiwi, lemon, mango, apple,
      melon, nectarine, pear, watermelon, grapes.
- Not advisable
    - Banana, strawberry, mandarine orange,
      honey melon, blackberry, oranges.

Legumes
- Beneficial
    - Facepiece beans, pinto beans
- Neutral
    - Kedney beans, garbanzo beans, green beans,
      peas, common lima beans.
- Not advisable
    - Lentils, white beans.

Vegetables
- Beneficial
    - Chard, garlic, marine alga, sweet potato,
      broccoli, pumpkin, onion, lettuce, turnip,
      parsley, red peppers, leeks.
- Neutral
    - Green olives, chives, asparagus, lime beans,
      fennel, cucumber, green peppers, radish,
      beet, tofu, tomatoes, carrot.
- Not advisable
    - Black olives, eggplant, cauliflower, Chinese
      cabbage, corn, avocado, potato, red cabbage,
      Brussels sprouts.

Spices
- Beneficial
    - Red algae, carrob tree, black algae, curry,
      parsley, cayenne pepper.

- Neutral
  - Agar, savory, garlic, basil, aniseed, arrow root, saffron, bergamot, clove, cumin, coriander, cream of tartar, chocolate, dill, almond essence, estragon, bay leafs, rice syrup, barley malt, marjoram, molasses, mint, maple syrup, mustard, paprika, pepper, radish, rosemary, sage, tamarind, tapioca, thyme.
- Not advisable
  - Capers, cornstarch, cinnamon, corn syrup, nutmeg, white pepper, ground black pepper, apple cider, vanilla, vinegar (all).

Infussions
- Beneficial
  - Fenugreek, cayenne, dandelion, ginger, hops, blackberry, elm, mint, parsley, rosehip, linden, sarsaparilla.
- Neutral
  - Birch, mullein, gingseng, chamomile, hawthorn, yarrow, white oak, sage, elder, green tea, thyme, valerian, verbena.
- Not advisable
  - Alfalfa, aloe, corn stubble, shepherd's bag, coltsfoot, gentian, St. John's wort, strawberry leaf, rhubarb, red clover.

GROUP "A" See
diet on page 95

They are descendants of the first farmers, and for this reason their diet is based on cereals, fish (almost all), fruit and chicken or turkey.   Their character is quiet, so they need less physical activity.

VERY HARMFUL FOOD (NEVER EAT IT)

Wheat, tomatoes, hake, garbanzo beans, lima beans, peppers, bananas, oranges, mandarins, pork, beef, lamb, potatoes, cow or goat milk.

COMMENTS

- Sugar is very harmful, we must restrain its intake. We must replace it by syrups or molasses.
- Tuna must be taken fresh or canned in olive oil.
- Take olive oil with moderation.
- Replace bread in lunch or dinner by whole wheat rice waffles or any other type of waffles. Or we can eat 25 gr. of spelt bread.

RECOMMENDED FOOD FOR GROUP "A"
Dairy products

☺Group A can tolerate small quantities of fermented dairy products, buy they should avoid all products elaborated with whole milk.

☹ Not advisable: Brie cheese, Camembert cheese, Emmental cheese, Gouda cheese, butter, Parmesan cheese, whole milk, Roquefort cheese and milk serum.

Nuts and seeds

☺ They can be a good source of vegetal protein. Advisable: Peanuts, pumpkin and sunflower seeds and peanut butter.

☹ Not advisable: Pistachios

Legumes

☺ Legumes provide a nutritious protein source which is very beneficial. Advisable: Peas, soy germ, lentils, black beans, kidney beans and green beans.

☹ Not advisable: Garbanzo beans and lima beans.

Meat

☺ It is advisable to replace meat by fish, and in any case, it is preferable to eat chicken to red meat.

☹ Not advisable: Duck, beef, pork, rabbit, liver, ham and bacon.

Fish

☺ People with group A can eat fish and seafood in moderate quantities, three of four times a week, they can take products like: Cod, mackerel, sea snails, mere, sardines, trout, salmon, perch, carp and golden fish.

☹ Not Advisable: Sole, halibut, pout, anchovies, eel, herring, squid, crab, caviar, mussels, hake, oysters and octopus.

Vegetables

☺Vegetables are very important for the diet of group A. Most vegetables are acceptable for this group, for example: Chard, garlic, artichoke, broccoli, onion, crisp cabbage, chicory, spinach, beet, lettuce, parsley, leek, radish, asparagus, cucumber, carrot and zucchini.

☹ But not advisable: Olives, sweet potatoes, lima beans, mushrooms, white or red potatoes, red or green peppers, white cabbage and tomatoes.

Fruits

☺Fruit is very beneficial for this group and they can take most fruits, for example: Black, green or red plums, dry or fresh figs, pineapple, persimmon, cherries, lemon, grapefruit, prines and grapes.

☹ But not advisable: Banana, coconut, mandarine orange, mango, melon, orange and papaya.

Drinks

☺ There are few drinks acceptable for Group A, for example: Mineral water, coffee, green tea, and red wine.

☹ But not advisable: Setz water, beer, soft drinks,

destilled liquors and black tea.

In our case, this diet done during eight weeks, followed by the letter, has given us great results.

After the eight weeks, if you want more variety in your diet, there are three factors to take into consideration:

1st.-See food recommendations explained before, and the list of foods indicated for each group on their corresponding chapter.

2nd.- Take into consideration some of the advise concerning foods to be avoided or reduced from Doctor Olga Cuevas:

- Fried food, eggs, asparagus, eggplant, spinach, beets, and peppers.
- Red meats, animal fat, sausages, dairy products (milk, cheese, yogurt, butter)
- Margarine.
- Sugar, honey, syrups and other sweeteners (to sweeten we can use a small quantity of molasses of rice or barley)
- All food that contains chemical products, dyes, pesticides or all products of chemical cultivation.
- Refined food and cereals and white flour.
- Strong spices, seasonings and exciting drinks.

3rd.-Follow a Mediterranean diet, in which fish prevails over meat, rich in fruit and with variety of vegetables, without forgetting carbohydrates. (pre-cooked brown rice, whole grain spelt wheat)

In our diet, we should try to include, twice a week, rice and spelt pasta.

We must consider salads very important, trying to eat them in all our meals, we recommend to include in them: lettuce, onion and carrots.

LIST OF FOODS FOR GROUP "A"

Grains and pasta
- Beneficial
  - Rice, rye, spelt and oatmeal flours, buckwheat, brown rice.
- Neutral
  - Barley flour, couscous, germinated wheat flour.
- Not advisable
  - Spinach pasta, semolina and wheat.

Bread
- Beneficial
  - Soy flour bread, rice waffles, Essene bread, Ezekiel bread, spelt bread.
- Neutral
  - Rice bread, Arabian bread, rye, millet, corn bread or rye toasts.
- Not advisable:
  - Multicereal bread, white bread, all bran bread.

Nuts
- Beneficial
    - Peanuts, pumpkin seeds, peanut butter.
- Neutral
    - Almonds, pine nuts, walnuts, sunflower seeds, hazelnuts, sesame, chestnuts.
- Not advisable
    - Pistachios, Brazilian nuts.

Meats
- Beneficial
    - None
- Neutral
    - Hen, turkey, chicken
- Not advisable (specially)
    - Buffalo, quail, partridge, duck, rabbit, bacon, beef, liver, pork, ham.

Fish and seafood
- Beneficial
    - Cod, mere, sardines, mackerel, perch, trout, carp, golden fish, sea trout, sturgeon.
- Neutral
    - Tuna, pike, sea bream, swordfish, halibut.
- Not advisable
    - Clams, shrimp, mussels, hake, anchovies, caviar, oysters, smoked salmon, herring, sole, octopus, turtle, scallop, squid, lobster.

Dairy products
- Beneficial
    - Rice and oatmeal milk.
- Neutral
    - Yogurt, goat cheese, sheep cheese, kefir.
- Not advisable

- Brie cheese, Camembert cheese, Gouda cheese, Gruyere cheese, Emmental cheese, Roquefort cheese, Edam or Swiss cheese, milk, butter, sorbet, serum.

Drinks
- Beneficial
    - Red wine, coffee, green tea.
- Neutral
    - White wine
- Not advisable
    - Sparkling water, beer, soda, cola, liquors.

Fruit
- Beneficial
    - Pineapple, apricot, grapefruit, cherry, fig, grapes, blackberry, blueberry, lemon, prunes, plums.
- Neutral
    - Persimmon, cranberry, melon, dates, guayaba, raisins, peach, kiwi, pear, raspberry, lime, watermelon, strawberry, apple, pomegranate, black or green grapes.
- Not advisable
    - Banana, mango, rhubarb, coconut, orange, mandarine orange, papaya, melon.

Legumes
- Beneficial
    - Peas, facepiece beans, soy, black beans, pinto beans, lentils.
- Neutral
    - Kidney beans, white beans and green beans.
- Not advisable
    - Garbanzo beans, red beans, lima beans, red beans.

Vegetables
- Beneficial
    - Chard, dandelion, leeks, garlic, chicory, radish, artichoke, spinach, carrot, broccoli, lettuce, lima beans, zucchini, onion, parsley, cauliflower.
- Neutral
    - Green olives, endive, avocado, algae, asparagus, cucumber, watercress, fennel, radish, mushrooms, beet, Chinese cabbage, Brussels sprouts.
- Not advisable
    - Black olives, white and red potatoes, sweet potatoes, lima beans, peppers, tomatoes, cabbage.

Cereals
- Beneficial
    - Buckwheat, amaranth, spelt.
- Neutral
    - Brown rice, corn flour, barley, all bran rice, millet, all bran oatmeal.
- Not advisable
    - Assorted cereals, all bran wheat, wheat germ, starch, granola, minced wheat.

Juices and liquids
- Beneficial
    - Pineapple juice, lemon juice, celery, plums, grapefruit, carrot, apricot, prune.
- Neutral
    - Apple juice, grape, cucumber, blueberry, apple cider.
- Not advisable
    - Orange juice, papaya and tomato.

Infussions

- Beneficial
  - Aloe, chamomile, alfalfa, rose hip, green tea, fenugreek, gingseng, valerian, barbana, hippuric.
- Neutral
  - Birch, shepperds bag, candelaria, dandelion, blackberry, gentian, green mint, peppermint, honey blanch, licorice, parsley, salvia, elder, lime-tree, thyme, verbena.
- Not advisable
  - Corn stubble, rhubarb, cayenne, red clover, catnip.

Spices

- Beneficial
  - Garlic, barley malt, ginger, soy sauce, millet mustard.
- Neutral
  - Agar, chives, nutmet, savory, clove, oregano, cumin, parsley, basil, sea weed, carob tree, cornstarch, saffron, corn flour, aniseed, cinnamon, cardamom, tartar cream, chocolate, tarragon, bay leaf, almond extract, non-refined rice syrup, mint, green mint, maple syrup, vanilla, honey, rosemary, tapioca.
- Not advisable
  - Capers, paprika, pepper, apple vinegar, ketchup, wine vinegar, mayonnaise, apple cider.

Seasonings

- Beneficial
  - Mustard.
- Neutral
  - Acid and sweet pickles, jelly, marmalade, sauces.
- Not advisable
  - Ketchup, mayonnaise, English sauce, vinegar (all).

GROUP "B" See
diet on page 95

They are a more evolved species, and they can eat more things, however, they are more delicate when eating chicken, corn, wheat and tomatoes.

Group B needs exercises which aren't too intense (like group "O") or too relaxed (like group "A", that is to say, they need moderate physical activity like walking, bike riding, tennis or aerobics.

VERY HARMFUL FOOD (NEVER EAT IT)
Wheat, tomotoes, bananas, chicken, lentils, peanuts, artichokes, coconut, persimmon, pomegranate, cow or goat milk.

COMMENTS
- Sugar is very harmful, its intake must be restricted. It must be replaced by syrup or molasses, with moderation.
- Tuna must be taken fresh or canned in olive oil.
- Olive oil must be taken in moderation.
- Replace bread on meals by brown rice wafers, or any other variety of wafers. Or by 25 gr. of spelt bread.

RECOMMENDED FOODS FOR GROUP "B"

Flours and pasta

☺ Group B doesn't need any excess in the use of these ingredients, they can use: oatmeal flour, rice flour, non-refined rice and spelt flour.

☹ But not advisable: rye flour, couscous, barley flour, whole wheat flour and gluten flour.

Dairy products

☺ Type B is the only one who can enjoy with a great variety of dairy products, but these products can also be replaced by products derived from soy. They can take: kefir, yogurt, goat cheese, sheep cheese, mozzarella. Oatmeal milk is very beneficial.

☹ Not advisable: ice cream, Roquefort cheese or melting cheese.

Nuts and seeds

☹ Most nuts and seeds are not advisable for the diet for type B. That's why they shouldn't take: hazelnuts, sunflower butter, pine seeds, pistachios, sunflower seeds, pumpkin seeds and sesame seeds.

Legumes

☺ There are few legumes tolerated by this group. Advisable: kidney beans, soy germ and white beans.

☹ But not advisable: garbanzo beans, lentils or facepiece beans.

Meats

☺Advisable: ram, lamb, rabbit and turkey.

☹ Not advisable: chicken, quail, pork, hen, ham and duck.

Fish

☺Type B pospers with nutrients and proteins coming from fish. Advisable: pout, cod, sea bream, mackerel, caviar, sole, hake, mere, perch, halibut, salmon and sardines.

☹ Not advisable: They must avoid all seafood, crab, lobster, shrimp, mussels, oysters, octopus and smoked salmon.

Vegetables

☺There is an enormous quantity of nutritive and high quality vegetables which are beneficial for this group, for example: garlic, sweet potato, eggplant, broccoli, pumpkin, onion, cauliflower, chicory, beet, lettuce, turnip, parsley, red pepper, leek, celery, watercress, asparagus, mushrooms, cucumber and carrot.

☹ Not advisable: olives, artichokes, corn, avocado and radish.

Fruits

☺There are very few fruits that should be avoided by group B, so they can eat delicious fruits like: pineapple, blueberry, banana, plums, papaya and grapes.

☹ Not advisable: persimmon, coconut, pomegranate and fig.

Drinks

☺ If they take tea, it will be neutral, but if they replace it by juice, green tea or other herbal infussions, they will notice how their efficiency is higher.

☹ Not advisable: Sparkling soft drinks, Seltz water and destilled liquors.

In our case, this diet done during eight weeks, followed by the letter, has given us great results.

After the eight weeks, if you want more variety in your diet, there are three factors to take into consideration:

1st.-See food recommendations explained before, and the list of foods indicated for each group on their corresponding chapter.

2nd.- Take into consideration some of the advise concerning foods to be avoided or reduced from Doctor Olga Cuevas:

- Fried food, eggs, asparagus, eggplant, spinach, beets, hand peppers.
- Red meats, animal fat, sausages, dairy products (milk, cheese, yogurt, butter)
- Margarine.

- Sugar, honey, syrups and other sweeteners
  (to sweeten we can use a small quantity of
  molasses of rice or barley)
- All food that contains chemical products,
  dyes, pesticides or all products of chemical
  cultivation.
- Refined food and cereals and white flour.
- Strong spices, seasonings and exciting drinks.

3rd.-Follow a Mediterranean diet, in which fish
prevails over meat, rich in fruit and with variety
of vegetables, without forgetting carbohydrates.
(pre-cooked brown rice, whole grain spelt wheat)

In our diet, we should try to include, twice a week, rice and spelt pasta.

We must consider salads very important, trying to eat them in all our meals, we recommend to include in them: lettuce, onion and carrots.

LIST OF FOODS FOR GROUP "B"

Grain and pasta
- Beneficial
  - Oatmeal flour, rice flour, spelt flour.
- Neutral
  - Spinach pasta, white rice, quinoa, brown rice.
- Not advisable
  - Rye flour, couscous, barley flour, wheat flour, whole wheat flour.

Bread

- Beneficial
    - Rice, millet, Essene, Ezekiel or spelt breads, rice waffles.
- Neutral
    - Soy bread, oatmeal bread, Arabian bread, pumpernickel.
- Not advisable
    - Rye bread, wheat bread, corn bread, multicereal bread, whole wheat bread.

Nuts

- Beneficial
    - None
- Neutral
    - Almonds, hazelnuts, chestnuts, walnuts
- Not advisable
    - Peanuts, pistachios, sunflower seeds, pumpkin seeds.

Meats

- Beneficial
    - Ram, rabbit, lamb, deer.
- Neutral
    - Pheasant, turkey, beef, cow, ham.
- Not advisable
    - Duck, partridge, chicken, bacon.

Fish and seafood

- Beneficial
    - Pout, cod, sea bream, mackerel, sturgeon, caviar, sole, pike, hake, mere, perch, halibut, salmon, sardines

- Neutral
    - Tuna, squid, carp, cazon, sturgeon, swordfish, trout, scallop.
- Not advisable
    - Clams, anchovies, eel, barracuda, shrimp, crab, sea snails, lobster, prawns, mussels, oysters, sea devil, octopus, frog, smoked salmon, turtle.

Dairy products
- Beneficial
    - Cottage cheese, kefir, yogurt, sheep cheese, mozzarella, goat cheese, ricotta cheese, oatmeal milk, rice milk.
- Neutral:
    - Brie cheese, Gouda cheese, butter, Gruyere cheese, Camembert cheese, Edam cheese, Emmenthal cheese, sorbet, soy cheese, soy milk.
- Not advisable
    - Ice cream, milk, cheddar cheese

Drinks
- Beneficial
    - Green tea
- Neutral
    - Beer, black tea, white wine, red wine.
- Not advisable
    - Seltz water, soda, cola, destilled liquors

Fruits
- Beneficial
    - Pineapple, banana, plums, grapes.
- Neutral
    - Cherries, apricots, dates, peach, raspberries,

    strawberries, figs, kiwi, lemon, mango, apple, mandarine orange, melon, nectarine, raisins, pears, grapefruit, prunes, watermelon.
- Not advisable
    - Persimmon, coconut, pomegranate, rhubarb.

Legumes
- Beneficial
    - Kidney beans, white beans, half moon beans.
- Neutral
    - Peas, green beans, red beans.
- Not advisable
    - Garbanzo beans, lentils, facepiece beans, black beans.

Vegetables
- Beneficial
    - Sweet potato, eggplant, cabbage, broccoli, Chinese cabbage, cauliflower, parsley, peppers, beet, Brussels sprouts, white cabbage, carrots.
- Neutral
    - Garlic, sea weeds, celery, watercress, pumpkin, onion, chicory, spinach, fennel, ginger, lettuce, turnip, potato, cucumber, leek, zucchini.
- Not advisable
    - Olives, artichokes, avocado, radish.

Cereals
- Beneficial
    - Crisp rice, spelt, millet, oatmeal flour, all bran rice and all bran oatmeal.
- Neutral
    - Rice cream, cornstarch, potato flour.

- Not advisable
    * Amaranth, barley, rye, wheat germ, wheat, corn flour, all bran wheat.

Juices and liquids
- Beneficial
    • Pineapple, blueberry, lemon, cabbage and grape juice.
- Neutral
    • Cider, apple, celery, plums, apricot, orange, cucumber, grapefruit, prune or carrot juice.
- Not advisable
    • Tomato juice.

Infussions
- Beneficial
    • Gingseng, ginger, licorice, mint, parsley, salvia.
- Neutral
    • Alfalfa, chamomile, green mint, green tea, thyme, valerian, verbena, sarsaparilla.
- Not advisable
    • Hops, rhubarb.

Spices
- Beneficial
    • Curry, ginger, parsley, hot radish.
- Neutral
    • Garlic, basil, capers, sea weeds, red algae, carob tree, aniseed, saffron, chives, chocolate, dill, bay leaf, mint, honey, mustard, oregano, paprika, rosemary, thyme, vanilla.
- Not advisable
    • Cinammon, jelly, cornstarch, barley malt, white and black pepper, tapioca.

Seasonings

- Beneficial
  - None
- Neutral
  - Sweet and sour pickles, jellies, mayonnaise, jam, mustard, English sauce.
- Not advisable
  - Ketchup

GROUP "AB"
See diet on page 95

They are a minority and they are the result of a mixture of groups A and B, so they have a mixture of positive and negative effects from both groups.

So, concerning physical exercise, they must combine the moderate activity of Group B with the relaxing activity of Group A.

VERY HARMFUL FOOD (NEVER EAT IT)

Wheat, garbanzo beans, peppers, banana, orange, artichoke, corn, hazelnuts, sunflower seeds, coconut, persimmon, chicken, cow or goat milk.

COMMENTS
- Sugar is very harmful, its intake must be restricted. It must be replaced by syrup or molasses, with moderation.
- Tuna must be taken fresh or canned in olive oil.
- Olive oil must be taken in moderation.
- Replace bread on meals by brown rice wafers, or any other variety of wafers. Or by 25 gr. of spelt bread.

RECOMMENDED FOODS FOR GROUP "AB"

Flours and pasta

🙂 In the diet for group AB, it is better to use rice to wheat, however, they are beneficial: rice, rice flour, oatmeal flour, rye flour, buckwheat flour, rice pasta and spinach pasta.   Spelt flour and other products derived from it are very advisable.

🙁 Not advisable: zobah noodles, buckwheat mush, and artichoke pasta.

Dairy products

😐 Dairy products can be taken with moderation, they can eat: kefir, mozzarella, sheep cheese, goat cheese, yogurt. Oatmeal milk is a good substitute for milk.

🙁 Not advisable: Camembert cheese, whole milk, butter, Brie cheese, Roquefort cheese and sorbet.

Nuts and seeds

😐 They are recommended to be taken in small quantities and with caution. Advisable: chestnuts, peanuts and walnuts.

🙁 But not advisable: hazel nuts, sunflower butter, sunflower seeds, sesame seeds and pumpkin seeds.

Legumes

🙂 This group can take an assorted range of legumes. Advisable: lentils, white beans, green beans and peas.

☹Not advisable: kidney beans, garbanzo beans and facepiece beans.

Meat

☺Group AB needs animal protein, advisable: lamb, turkey, rabbit or ram.

☹Not advisable: pork, ham, duck, chicken, beef, bacon.

Fish

☺There is a big variety of fish for this group, and besides they are excellent source of proteins. Advisable: cod, sea bream, mackerel, hake,
mere, perch, salmon, sardine and trout..

☹ Not advisable:pout, herring, clams, shrimp, crab, oysters, octopus, halibut and smoked salmon.

Vegetables

☺People of group AB can choose from a varied range of products which will provide them with lots of benefits. Advisable: garlic, celery, sweet potato, broccoli, cauliflower, cucumber, parsley, cabbage, beets and peas.

☹ Not advisable: olives, corn, pepper and radish.

Fruits

☺They follow trends of Group A, so they are beneficial: pineapple, blueberries, cherrie`s, plums, figs, kiwi, lemon, grapefruit and grapes.

☹ Not advisable: banana, persimmon, coconut, pomegranate, mango and oranges.

Drinks

☺ Beneficial for group AB are: green tea, mineral water, beer, white wine and red wine.

☹ Not advisable: sparkling soft drinks, destilled liquors and black tea.

In our case, this diet done during eight weeks, followed by the letter, has given us great results.

After the eight weeks, if you want more variety in your diet, there are three factors to take into consideration:

1st.-See food recommendations explained before, and the list of foods indicated for each group on their corresponding chapter.

2nd.- Take into consideration some of the advise concerning foods to be avoided or reduced from Doctor Olga Cuevas:

- Fried food, eggs, asparagus, eggplant, spinach, beets, and peppers.
- Red meats, animal fat, sausages, dairy products (milk, cheese, yogurt, butter)
- Margarine.
- Sugar, honey, syrups and other sweeteners (to sweeten we can use a small quantity of molasses of rice or barley)

- All food that contains chemical products, dyes, pesticides or all products of chemical cultivation.
- Refined food and cereals and white flour.
- Strong spices, seasonings and exciting drinks.

3rd.-Follow a Mediterranean diet, in which fish prevails over meat, rich in fruit and with variety of vegetables, without forgetting carbohydrates. (pre-cooked brown rice, whole grain spelt wheat)

In our diet, we should try to include, twice a week, rice and spelt pasta.

We must consider salads very important, trying to eat them in all our meals, we recommend to include in them: lettuce, onion and carrots.

LIST OF FOODS FOR GROUP "AB"

Grains and pasta
- Beneficial
  - Basmati rice, brown rice, white rice, rice flour, oatmeal and germinated rye.
- Neutral
  - Couscous, flour gluten, semolina noodles, barley, spelt and quinoa flour.
- Not advisable
  - Zhoba noodles, wheat mush, artichoke pasta.

Bread
- Beneficial
    - Millet bread, rice waffles, Essene bread, Ezekiel bread, rice bread, spelt bread, rye bread, soy bread.
- Neutral
    - Arabian bread, bread without gluten, oatmeal, acimo bread.
- Not advisable
    - Corn bread.

Cereals
- Beneficial
    - Crisped rice, millet, oatmeal, all bran rice and all bran oatmeal.
- Neutral
    - Amaranth, barley, starch, rice cream, granola, wheat germ, soy granules.
- Not advisable
    - Corn flour, buckwheat, corn mush, corn

Nuts
- Beneficial
    - Chestnuts, peanuts, peanut butter, walnuts.
- Neutral
    - Almonds, pine seeds, pistachios.
- Not advisable
    - Hazelnuts, sunflower butter, sunflower seeds, sesame seeds, pumpkin seeds.

Meat
- Beneficial
    - Ram, rabbit, lamb, turkey.
- Neutral
    - Liver, pheasant.

- Not advisable
    - Buffalo, pork, quail, bacon, heart, hen, goose, deer, duck, chicken, partridge, beef.

Fish and seafood
- Beneficial
    - Tuna, cod, sea bream, mackerel, sea snails, sturgeon, pike, mere, hake, perch, shad, salmon, sardine, trout.
- Neutral
    - Caviar, shark, herring, squid, swordfish, mussels, carp, sole.
- Not advisable
    - Clams, crab, anchovies, barracuda, oysters, eel, lobster, shrimp, prawns, octopus, smoked salmon, halibut.

Dairy products
- Beneficial
    - Kefir, mozzarella, eggs, goat cheese, sheep cheese.
- Neutral
    - Emmenthal cheese, Suisse cheese, Gouda cheese, Edam cheese, Gruyere cheese and soy milk.
- Not advisable
    - Roquefort cheese, parmesan cheese, Brie cheese, Camembert cheese, ice cream, milk, butter, sorbet.

Drinks
- Beneficial
    - Green tea, red tea.
- Neutral
    - White wine, red wine, mineral water and beer.

- Not advisable
    • Soda, cola, diet drinks, black tea, liquors.

Juices and liquids
- Beneficial
    • Celery, carrot, blueberry, papaya, cherry, and grape juice.
- Neutral
    • Apple cider, pineapple, plums, apricot, apple, cucumber, grapefruit juices.
- Not advisable
    • Orange juice.

Fruit
- Beneficial
    • Pineapple, cherry, fig, blueberry, plums, cranberry, grape, kiwi, lemon, grapefruit.
- Neutral
    • Apricot, dates, peach, raspberry, strawberry, lime, melon, mandarine orange, apple, honey melon, blackberry, papaya, raisin, pear, prune, elder, watermelon, blackberry.
- Not advisable
    • Banana, persimmon, coconut, pomegranate, guayaba, mango, orange, rhubarb.

Legumes
- Beneficial
    • Lentils, white beans, soy, red beans.
- Neutral
    • Peas, green beans, red lentils.
- Not advisable
    • Kidney beans, garbanzo beans, facepiece beans, half moon beans, pinto beans.

Vegetables
- Beneficial
    - Garlic, celery, sweet potato, cabbage, broccoli, cauliflower, alfalfa sprouts, parnsnip, dandelion, cucumber, parsley, beet, tofu, soy.
- Neutral
    - Green olives, chard, algae, watercress, bamboo, Chinese cabbage, onion, mushroom, pumpkin, kohlrabi, coriander, endives, chicory, asparagus, spinach, fennel, tomato, ginger, lettuce, potatoe, leek, radish, Brussels sprouts, carrot, zucchini.
- Not advisable
    - Black olives, artichokes, radish sprouts, corn, avocado, radish, green pepper, yellow pepper.

Spices
- Beneficial
    - Soy oil, garlic, parsley, curry, hot radish
- Neutral
    - Agar, savory, Moorish garlic, basil, carob tree, cinnamon, chocolate, dill, tarragon, soy sauce, thyme, saffron, bay leaf, marjoram, mint, honey, sage, clove, vanilla, cumin, mustard, nutmeg, rosemary, paprika, tamarind, pepper.
- Not advisable
    - Spicy chilli, capers, cornstarch, aniseed, gelatine, almond extract, malt, pepper, tapioca, all vinegars.

Infussions
- Beneficial
    - Alfalfa, burdock, rose hip, ginseng, strawberry leaf, chamomile, ginger, marjolato, licorice, green tea, red tea.

- Neutral
    - Birch, raspberry, elm, cayenne, dandelion, hypericum, honey branch, thyme, valerian, mint, sage, elder, parsley.
- Not advisable
    - Fenugreek, aloe, corn stubble, candelaria, escufelaria, gentian, hops, rhubarb, sena, lime, red clover.

MARTA'S ADVISE

Besides doing this diet, it is convenient to follow this advise that has been so useful to Marta.

- Its convenient to sunbathe (with moderation, ten to fifteen minutes) during the summer, avoiding strong hours of sun rays.
- Its important to do some exercise regularly, each person must practice an adequate activity according to his physical and mental condition.
- During meals, we can eat brown rice waffles.
- During the first weeks of diet, it's advisable to accompany it with physiotherapy.
- It's recommended the intake of licorice, with moderation (in pills or natural) because it helps to detoxify the liver.
- Nutrition is a new science in constant evolution, which together with traditional medicine will bring an important medical revolution in the XXI century.
- I also wish to warn you about the harmful effects of coffee and tobacco on this disease.

COFFEE

Coffee is the most popular stimulating drink taken in Spain. Each cup of coffee contains between 75 and 150 mg of caffeine. With this dosage, caffeine has a stimulating action on our central nervous system, which, on most sensitive people, can be prolonged several hours and produce insomnia.

Coffee is a heart stimulant, and in sensitive people, or in high dosage, it can produce heart palpitations and tachycardia. In addition, it acts on our blood vessels reducing their size, and favouring hypertension. Couriously, this effect, generally harmful for our health, is also the one that causes headache disappearance.

Its intake, after meals, helps with digestion because caffeine activates stomach fluids and bowel movements. This is what causes some people to have heartburn and/or diarrhea, or simply produces a laxative or diuretic effect.

Tolerance to coffee is very different from one person to another, but it should be totally removed from our diet in the following cases: insomnia, cystitis, hypertension, heartburn, diarrhea, ulcerative colitis or other bowel disorders.

Decaffeinated coffee in big quantities becomes toxic, due to the waste left by the chemical thinner used in the process of decaffeination. But, in return, it doesn't have the stimulating effects of caffeine. Coffee can be replaced by ginger, green tea... always the ones allowed for our blood group.

TOBACCO

We could consider it as one of the most harmful drugs for our health, considering that to the many harmful effects it produces on our bodies, we must add that it creates addiction (we need enormous willpower and external help to abandon it), and it can affect us even if we don't smoke because, for the time being, smoking is still allowed in jobs and public places.

According to   Dr. Olga Cuevas, the harmful components of tobacco and smoke are:

- Nicotine, a substance that causes dependence, which makes it responsible for many behavioral disorders (anxiety, nervousness, fatigue and irritability).
- Tars, some with cancerous effects.
- Carbon monoxide, which alters our oxygen uptake causing injuries on our heart tissues.
- It can affect our breathing, it produces headaches, it leads to acne, it favours hair loss, it makes our teeth yellow and it tightens our blood vessels.

And the diseases associated to smoking are many:

- Affecting our nervous system, like memory and vision disorders.
- Lung, larynx, bladder and stomach cancer.
- Chronic bronchitis, emphysema.
- It causes arterial tightening, heart diseases, and it produces gastric ulcers.

Recipes

SPELT PIZZA WITH ONION
Ingredients:

Pizza base
Onion
Sheep cheese
Turkey ham
Olive oil

How to prepare:
Cut and chop the onion, the quantity to your taste, stir fry and when golden put on top of the pizza base.

Cut the sheep cheese and the turkey ham and put it on top.

Put it in the oven 10 minutes approximately.

VEGETABLE PIZZA
Ingredients:

Pizza base
Allowed vegetables for each group (see list)
Sheep cheese
Olive oil

How to prepare:
Cut the vegetables in small pieces, cook them in a pan with a bit of oil and water, stir until done.
Extend then on top of the pizza base adding the cut or grated cheese.

Put in the oven 10 minutes approximately.

PASTA WITH BROCCOLI
Ingredients:

Rice or spelt pasta (spirals, macaroni, spaghetti)
Broccoli
Sheep cheese
Olive oil
Tuna (low in salt)
Onion

How to prepare:
Boil pasta in water and salt (rice pasta about 15 minutes, and spelt pasta from 8 to 10 minutes)

Cut onion and broccoli and stir fry with oil and water.

When done, add the pasta and mix together.

Serve in a plate putting on top some grated sheep cheese and tuna.

**LENTILS WITH VEGETABLES
Ingredients:**

Dry or canned lentils
Onion, carrot, leek, potato (except groups "O" and "A")
Olive oil
Precooked brown rice
Algae
Salt

How to prepare:
Put all together in a pot cut in small pieces, and cook.

Twenty minutes before ending the cooking process, add the precooked brown rice and some algae, oil and salt.

Cook until done to our taste.

**BEANS WITH ALGAE AND RICE
Ingredients:**

Beans (Dry or canned)
Algae
Precooked brown rice
Salt
Olive oil
Potato
Onion

How to prepare:
Put beans in a pot, if canned add to them the precooked rice, algae, oil and salt.

If they are dry, cook them first with onion and potato (except groups "O" and "A") for some time, and twenty minutes before the end of the cooking process, add the precooked rice, algae, oil and salt.

Finish the cooking during twenty more minutes and serve.

MACARONI WITH BECHAMEL SAUCE
Ingredients:

Rice or spelt macaroni
Milk (better of soy or oatmeal)
Olive oil
Salt
Onion
Tuna
Rice or spelt flour
Sheep cheese

How to prepare:
Boil pasta in water and salt (15 minutes for rice pasta and 8 to 10 for spelt pasta)

Grate the onion and fry in oil, add flour and stir. Add

milk, of oatmeal or soy, stir so it doesn't stick, when the béchamel sauce is done, add the pasta and mix together.

Serve with grated cheese and tuna.

TURKEY SAUSAGES WITH VEGETABLES
Ingredients:

Turkey sausages
Onion
Red pepper
Olive oil
Pumpkin
Salt

How to prepare:
Cut vegetables in small pieces, and then fry in a bit of oil, stirring to avoid burning them.

Cut sausages in small pieces and then add to the frying.

When done, we can serve.

RICE AND PEAS SALAD
Ingredients:

Precooked brown rice
Peas

Olive oil
Salt
Tuna
Mayonnaise

How to prepare:
Boil the pre-cooked rice during 20 minutes in water, salt and oil.

Rinse it with cold water, to avoid sticking.

When cold, add peas, tuna and a bit of salt.

We can add some mayonnaise, better homemade and without vinegar.

Serve cold.

POTATO AND PUMPKIN
Ingredients:

Potatoes
Pumpkin, zucchini
Onion
Red pepper
Tomato
Olive oil
Water
Salt

How to prepare:
Cut all ingredients in small pieces and put them in a deep pan with oil and salt.

Add water and stir from time to time.

It must turn out to be like a mush.

MILLET WITH CAULIFLOWER OR BROCCOLI
Ingredients:

Millet
Broccoli or cauliflower
Olive oil
Salt
Algae

How to prepare:
Fry grated onion in olive oil.

Add millet, algae and water. The proportion is one of millet and two of water.

Boil during 15 or 20 minutes.

Serve warm.

TURKEY MEATBALLS WITH POTATOES
Ingredients:

Five turkey meatballs per person-
Olive oil (two tablespoons)
Potatoes
Salt
Parsley

How to prepare:
Fry in a pan or pot the meatballs with two tablespoons of olive oil, with low heat.

When they are a little bit golden, add potatoes cut up in stripes, just like for French fries.

Add water and a bit of salt.

Cook until potatoes are done and serve.

PORK LOIN WITH ALMONDS
Ingredients:

Two "books" of pork loin per person
Olive oil
Toasted and crushed almonds
Milk
Salt

How to prepare:
Put almonds inside the books.

Fry them in oil (not much) and when golden, take them out. Put the books in a big pot, better made of clay, and add the milk. When it starts boiling, add the rest of the almonds. It will be ready when the sauce thickens.

Note: This dish may also be prepared with turkey and soy milk.

PUMPKIN BISCUIT
Ingredients:

1 glass of oatmeal, soy or rice milk
1 glass of all bran spelt flour
1 egg (it can be done without it)
2 tablespoons of rice molasses
2 tablespoons of maple syrup
2 tablespoons of olive oil
1 teaspoon of baking soda
1 Kg of sweet pumpkin (previously cooked in the oven)

How to prepare:
Put all ingredients in a bowl.

Beat them and put them in a deep tray, greased with oil.

Put in the oven until it gets hard and toasted. It will turn out to be like a creamy pudding and it is delicious. Serve cold.

Keep it in the fridge.

Note: This biscuit can also be done replacing pumpkin with raisins, figs or apple. Apple must be pealed cut, and beat together with the other ingredients.

AGUARDIENTE (LIQUOR) COOKIES
Ingredients:

One glass of olive oil
Half glass of aguardiente (liquor)
All bran spelt flour and brown rice flour
Agave syrup or rice molasses

How to prepare:
Put in a bowl the oil and the aguardiente, with rice molasses or syrup, mix well add flour, half of each type, and knead. It must turn out to be a bit hard, extend and give form, better with a mold.

Author

My name is Maribel, and I want to tell you my story.

I was born on the 13th March 1967 in a beautiful family, I have three more sisters, I'm the oldest.

I remember my childhood and teenage years with pains all over my body, specially on my wrists, feet and back. Besides, I always suffered with intestinal gases and frequent diarrhea. If I tell you the truth, I never thought I would solve these problems, I thought it was normal to feel that way each day.

I had to wait until the birth of my second daughter to start looking for solutions.

Marta was born on the 29th December 1990.

When she was only three years old, she was already diagnosed with irritable bowel, just like me. But Marta's problems started when she was three, and she started having pains on her heels. Through the years, other pains were added on her knees, back, hands, neck... and on to her whole little body. She was eleven years old when she was diagnosed with severe teenage fibromyalgia and chronic fatigue, after years of specialist not knowing what was the cause of her terrible pain.

That diagnose was the triggering reason for the quest started by her father and I, just so we could get our daughter out of that pain that nobody knew how to explain, WHAT IS IT? WHY DOES IT APPEAR? HOW CAN IT BE CURED?

We started looking for information and it came in the most unsuspected ways, books and experiences that opened our eyes to a new world, the world of NUTRITION, and how with an appropriate nutrition we can prevent and cure diseases.

We have explained all these studies accomplished by the most important physicians and nutritionists of the moment during ten years, we have published two books containing our work on hundreds of patients, and now from this blog, we want to help patients all over the world.

Sometimes, fate has something prepared for us that we ignore, which might be the reason why we came to this world. We all have a mission in life, and we believe ours is to expand our knowledge and help patients like Marta to recover their health and the happiness of living without pain. This is my story, and the story of thousands of patients like you.

You can change your life. These books are fruit of my sleeplessness, my experience, my trials.

These books can help you to recover your health. Through these years, we have tried different ways of nutrition, different foods that might benefit Marta as well as other patients. No patient is identical, each person has his own beneficial and harmful food. On these books, I'll teach you how to distinguish them.

But, the most important thing in these books is that I HAVE SUFFERED THE DISEASE MYSELF, in my case it is Candidas. Other therapists may think they know how much pain the patient is going through, but they have never experienced that pain. I have suffered it personally, I perfectly understand the patient, I have been a patient myself. I know about the pain, about his doubts, about the suffering caused by the incomprehension at home.

As I said before, I have suffered the pain since I was very little, but it was now until one year after following Marta's therapy (all my family decided to eat like her, just to give her full support), that I noticed that my pain on hands, feet, head,... were gone, and it was a big surprise. At that moment I thought "I have always suffered fibromyalgia", but no, my diagnose is not fibromyalgia, it is Candidas. The symptoms are the same.

That is the reason why I always treat my patients with a diet suitable for Candidas.

Before I started with the therapy, my life was quite complicated. I always had pain on some part of my body. It was a trauma even preparing a nice vacation for the family, the pain, the fatigue, and my bad mood came out only by preparing the suitcase, everything became a terrible trial full of stress for me. I was never able to enjoy a vacation. Now, it's not a problem for me to prepare a suitcase.

I've written these books to help you, just so you can feel understood, and so you understand why you suffer this pain. You are not alone, like your doctor and family are telling you. I'm on your side to help you in this travel that will take you to enjoying your life and your family again.

REMEMBER

You are the only one who has the power over yourself. You are the one to decide how you want to spend the rest of your life.

SOMETHING VERY IMPORTANT

You can send me and e-mail to get in contact with me. You can express your doubts, I will answer you. You can also tell me your story is you wish to do so.

In my blog and in my books, you will find answers to your questions:

WHAT IS IT?, WHY DOES IT APPEAR?, AND HOW TO CONTROL FIBROMYALGIA , ALL ITS SYMPTOMS AND ALL DISEASES THAT COME WITH IT?

www.comidasana.eu
info@comidasana.eu